FOODWISE

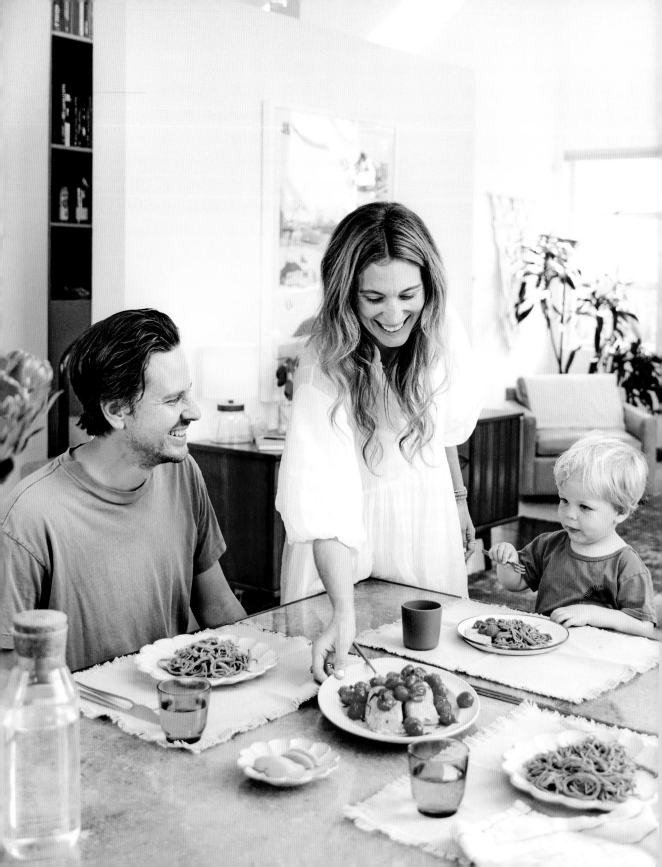

FOODWISE

A FRESH APPROACH TO NUTRITION WITH 100 DELICIOUS RECIPES

MIA RIGDEN

SIMON ELEMENT
NEW YORK   LONDON   TORONTO   SYDNEY   NEW DELHI

SIMON
ELEMENT

An Imprint of Simon & Schuster, Inc.
1230 Avenue of the Americas
New York, NY 10020

First Simon Element hardcover edition January 2023

SIMON ELEMENT and colophon are trademarks of Simon & Schuster, Inc.

For information about special discounts for bulk purchases, please contact Simon
& Schuster Special Sales at 1-866-506-1949 or business@simonandschuster.com.

The Simon & Schuster Speakers Bureau can bring authors to your live event.
For more information or to book an event, contact the Simon & Schuster Speakers
Bureau at 1-866-248-3049 or visit our website at www.simonspeakers.com.

Interior design by Matt Ryan
Photography by Andrew Purcell
Food styling by Carrie Purcell

Manufactured in China

3 5 7 9 10 8 6 4 2

Library of Congress Cataloging-in-Publication Data has been applied for.

ISBN 978-1-9821-8238-0
ISBN 978-1-9821-8239-7 (ebook)

To Jamie,
my hype man, taste tester
& forever Reset partner.
I love you.

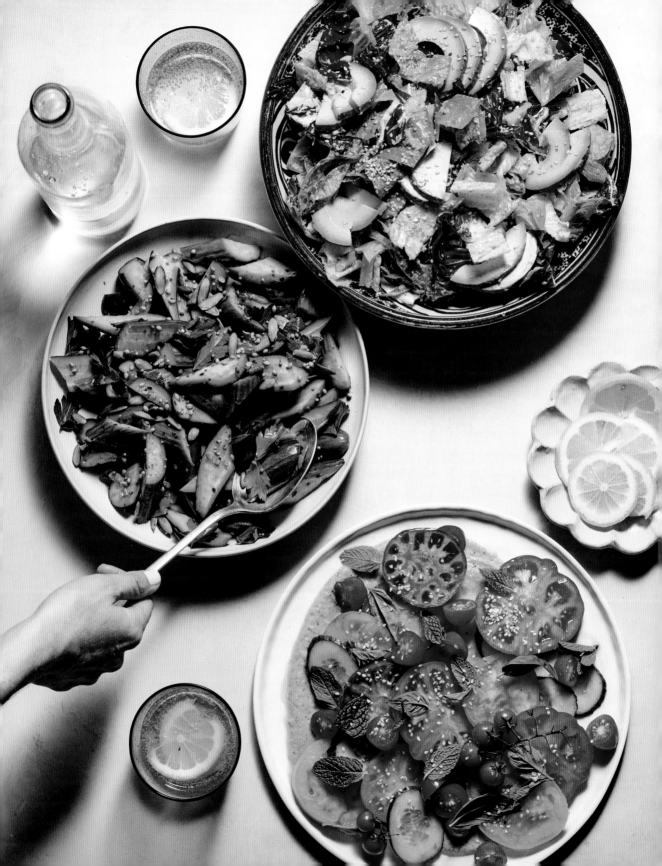

Contents

Smoothies & Breakfast

Mint–Chocolate Chip Smoothie **93**

Sesame-Cardamom Smoothie **93**

Cucumber-Vanilla Smoothie **95**

Pumpkin Pie Smoothie **95**

Supreme Green Smoothie **96**

Golden Smoothie **98**

Raspberry-Beet Smoothie **98**

Chocolate-Covered Cherry Smoothie **99**

Blueberry-Basil Smoothie **99**

Garlicky Kale Frittata **100**

Almond-Banana Pancakes **103**

Grain-Free Hot Cereal **103**

Vegetables & Salads

Roasted Cauliflower with Popcorn Capers, Pine Nuts & Tahini Dressing **106**

Miso Caesar Salad **107**

Green Goddess Salad **109**

Winter Citrus Salad with Crispy Shallots **110**

Roasted Sunchokes with Lotsa Herbs **113**

Spicy Roasted Broccoli Rabe **114**

Turmeric Cauliflower **115**

Purple Sweet Potato Fries **116**

Sesame Broccoli Poppers **119**

Spiced Carrot Salad **120**

Warm Chicory Salad **121**

Hot & Cold Cucumber Salad **122**

Simple Green Salad **124**

Eggplant Caponata **125**

Heirloom Tomato, Sesame & Herb Salad with Green Miso Dressing **127**

Quinoa & Arugula Salad **128**

Meal-Prep Roasted Vegetables **129**

Rainbow Chop with Carrot-Ginger Dressing **130**

Mixed Green Salad with Ginger, Carrots & Mulberries **132**

Celery, Fennel, & Apple Salad **133**

Noodles & Grains

Lemongrass Black Rice **135**

Spiced Quinoa Cakes **137**

Socca Flatbread **138**

Herbed Brown Rice & Cauliflower Pilaf **139**

Mushrooms & Fonio **141**

Super Green Spaghetti with Zucchini Pesto **142**

Chicken, Peanut & Soba Noodle Salad **144**

Fusilli with Braised Chicken Thighs, Mushrooms, Spinach & Sun-Dried Tomato Pesto **145**

Fresh Crab & Arugula Spaghetti **147**

Shrimp & Veggie Pad Thai **148**

Meat, Poultry & Seafood

Chimichurri Steak Salad with Chickpea Croutons **151**

Turkey Lettuce Wraps **152**

Zaatar-Crusted Chicken Cutlets with Arugula Salad **155**

Chicken en Papillote **156**

Herbed Leg of Lamb **157**

Shepherd's Pie with Celery Root Top **158**

Spiced Chicken with Green Olives **161**

Mediterranean Lamb Meatball Lettuce Wraps **162**

Grilled Skirt Steak Piled with Shiitake Mushrooms & Onions **163**

Spaghetti with Caramelized Onions, Collard Greens & Bacon **164**

Harissa Salmon **165**

Salmon Niçoise **167**

Spiced Tomato & Shrimp Bisque **168**

Coconut-Saffron Mussels **171**

Cod Puttanesca **172**

Roasted Salmon with Cherry Tomatoes & Shallots **175**

Soup

Snacks, Sweets & Baked Goods

Elevated Pantry Essentials

Nut & Seed Milks

Hydration Station

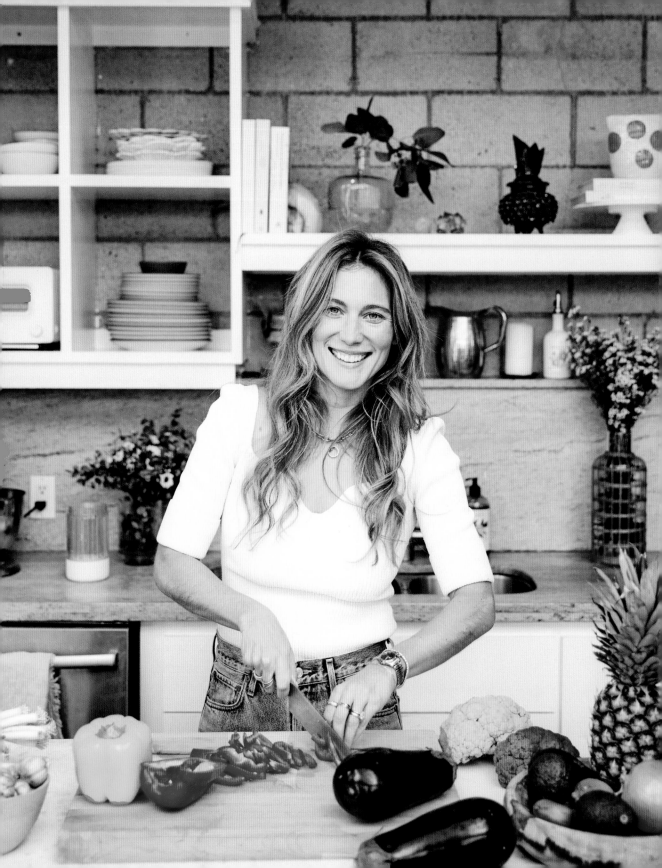

This is not your typical "eat this, don't eat that" diet book. In fact, this is not a diet book at all. So, if you're looking for that magic bullet or empty promises of flat abs in two weeks, let me be clear: You will not find that here.

What you will find, however, is a path toward food freedom, reconnecting with your taste buds, and feeling great in the body you were born with.

Hi, I'm Mia Rigden, a board-certified nutritionist and professionally trained chef. The principles and philosophies found in this book are the result of years of client work and postgraduate studies, as well as my personal experience. My journey began with food. Everyone in my family cooks; both my parents are excellent cooks, and my grandmother was not only the queen of pumpkin pie and roast chicken, but was also an ardent student of nutrition. She studied at Carnegie Mellon in the 1930s and was always ahead of her time, cooking with and slathering coconut oil all over herself in the 1990s when popular nutrition culture wouldn't touch fat with a ten-foot pole.

I started working in restaurants when I was fifteen. First as a host, then a server, and after college I moved to New York and enrolled at The French Culinary Institute (now part of the Institute for Culinary Education). I had an exciting career in restaurant public relations, during which I worked with some of the top restaurants and chefs in the city. It was a twenty-five-year-old's dream: free meals and choice reservations at all the hot spots. I loved it, until I didn't. At some point, all the dining out (and let's be honest, going out) took its toll. I had gained weight and felt off, so I started to experiment with different cleanses, diets, and fitness programs. I was constantly oscillating from periods of extreme healthy eating to indulgent nights out for work and with friends. I loved how I felt when I was eating "clean," but that rigidity was at odds with my career and my social life, and I couldn't figure out how to align those forces.

A chance encounter at a friend's roller derby disco birthday party in New York City introduced me to my husband, Jamie, a charming Brit with an expiring visa. He was unable to stay in the United States, so his company transferred him to Hong Kong, and I went with him. Leaving the hustle in New York gave me the time and space to hone my passion for nutrition and cooking while I traveled throughout Asia, learning about the cultures and traditions of the East.

I went to India right around the time I finished the first part of my nutrition education—a health-coaching certification program from the Institute for Integrative Nutrition. Cliché, I know, but stick with me. One lazy afternoon after a morning of sightseeing in a small village outside Jaipur, I was lounging by the hotel pool reading Deepak Chopra's *Perfect Health* and came across *rasa*, a Sanskrit word that has many meanings, but among them, "taste." In Ayurveda, the concept of taste has so much more depth than the way it's commonly used in the West; taste is the essence of life. Different flavors are indicative of a food's nutritional properties and can be used to create harmony in both our physical and spiritual bodies. When I read this, a light bulb went off. Everything I had been taught about dieting and wellness was through the lens of restriction, sacrifice, and compromise. It was the angel and the devil on my shoulder, and I didn't think it was possible to have it both ways. As an avid cook and food lover, I struggled with this and had developed an unhealthy relationship with food as a result, but I realized I had it backward; **nutrition is about taste**. Our body is constantly giving us feedback, we just need to listen to what it is trying to tell us and learn how to respond.

I went on to get a masters in nutrition and integrative health, then became a board-certified nutritionist. In my client work, I aim to help people find that alignment between their actions and their goals, and figure out how to apply nutrition science to their everyday lives in a way that feels sustainable and, dare I say, fun.

Many of my clients come to me fighting through fatigue, constant bloating, headaches, skin issues, food sensitivities, stubborn weight gain, chronic stress, and more. They have tried it all, from paleo and keto to meticulous macro counting, vegan, and carnivore; and spent hundreds—if not thousands—of dollars on supplements, books, fitness programs, and meal-delivery services. And while they may have had some level of temporary success trying different programs, they weren't able to stick with it and definitely didn't enjoy it. Frustrated, exhausted, and confused, they end up in my office searching for a different approach.

So how do you get to the place where you can eat what you want, weigh what you want, and feel amazing? Well, this is precisely what you're going to learn in this book. Let me break it down for you.

In order to align our taste buds with what our body truly needs, we have to do a little self-discovery. As you learn more about how what you eat affects other areas of your life (like your mood, sleep, energy, and stress levels), you will be more in control of how you feel and naturally gravitate toward food and activities that are supportive of your body.

A few years back, I was working with a client who had gained about twenty pounds since starting a career in finance, had low energy, consistent bloating, and just wasn't feeling herself. In our first session, she pleaded, "Please don't take my bagel from me."

I assured her that I wouldn't, but suggested she try out some other breakfasts just to see how they would feel. She went three weeks without her beloved bagel fix, until one Friday morning a colleague of hers ordered some in for the office. She thought, *I've been so good, I deserve this!* and went for it.

Later that afternoon she emailed me, saying she had felt tired and bloated all day. She started to question whether she even liked bagels and cream cheese anymore. I replied, "Well, this might be the best bagel you've ever had."

Why? Because I didn't have to tell her that a food she loved was keeping her from her goals; her relationship with the food changed instinctively. It wasn't a battle of good and bad; she didn't have to start each day with guilt about what she had for breakfast, or feel unsatisfied by her "healthy" choice. This simply became a personal preference. Now, does this mean she hates bagels and will never have them again? Absolutely not! But a once-everyday food became an occasional food, and switching to a nutrient-dense breakfast changed her whole day: She went from feeling tired, bloated, and craving sugar, to feeling energized, satisfied, and proud of her food choices. What a win!

We all have our own version of a bagel and cream cheese—a food or activity that we know isn't getting us any closer to our goals, but for some reason we can't shake. Diet culture says, "Don't eat bagels," but in my experience, we have to get to the why if we want to be successful in making a change. Telling someone not to eat something because it's "bad" isn't so convincing. When you can see, feel, taste, and truly understand the difference, food preferences take on a whole new meaning, and consistency becomes easy. This is food freedom, and it comes from being food wise.

Set Your New Baseline with The Reset

The Reset (detailed in part 2) is a twenty-one-day whole foods plan that will help you find the most supportive foods and routines for your body and learn how to integrate them into your everyday life. In this program, we remove common food sensitivities and dependencies—like gluten, dairy, alcohol, and sugar—so you can gain a deeper understanding of how they affect your body, while giving your gut a chance to heal, and allowing you to reconnect with your natural energy and find new habits you can easily continue after your Reset is complete.

After completing The Reset, you'll have a clean slate onto which you can carefully and intentionally reintroduce foods and monitor how they make you feel. You may find that foods you used to eat regularly taste really sweet or make you feel off. For example, when you reintroduce gluten, do you feel bloated, tired, or anxious? Maybe you will, and maybe you won't! The most exciting part of The Reset is not what you accomplish in the twenty-one days, but how it helps shape your food and lifestyle preferences moving forward. Here is some real client feedback I've received over the years:

"I now eat nutritiously because I want to, not because I need to."

"I lost fourteen pounds, was getting amazing sleep, my acne cleared up, and I was generally much happier. The craziest thing was that I didn't feel I was making drastic sacrifices."

"The program was the first time I not only made progress, but it also felt sustainable, which to me is a big deal."

"I feel really, really good. Sleeping so well, my skin is better than it's been in years, I feel like I experience hunger in a totally different way, which I would have rolled my eyes at twenty-one days ago."

"I no longer get those growly stomachs at four p.m. that come with a mad lust for sugar and an energy crash."

"I have become so much more in tune with my body and its reactivity to certain foods."

"My skin is glowing, and normally in the winter it feels so dull and dry."

"I have lost weight, which is really good news, as I have hypothyroidism and haven't been able to lose an ounce in three years."

"I cannot believe the difference in my skin, especially those bags under my eyes."

Invariably, over time, small things start to creep back in, like sugar, alcohol, excess coffee, or processed snacks, but when my clients start to feel tired, or out of their groove, they know exactly what to do to turn things around. Your wellness journey will not be linear; you might take two steps forward, then one step back, or perhaps you move, change jobs, have children, or experience other life events that affect your routines, but you'll find yourself in a more comfortable space than when you started and have the tools to get back on track. It only takes twenty-one days.

If this sounds simple to you, that's because it is! This isn't about restriction, it's about approaching our relationship to food with a more dynamic definition of taste. And while your truth might be hiding in plain sight, I'm not going to sugarcoat it for you; there's work involved. So, before we get started, I want to establish a few ground rules:

Be open to having your mind changed. There are many beliefs when it comes to nutrition that we need to let go of. Plus, the field of nutrition science is constantly evolving, and sometimes new research comes out that contradicts what we previously thought was true. For example, we now know that eggs have been exonerated as a driver for high cholesterol and that fat is good for you!

Healthy does not equal skinny. It's okay to want to feel great in your body and confident when you look in the mirror, but let's not confuse health with unrealistic weight goals. Healthy people come in all shapes and sizes, and first and foremost, this book is about health. You may very well lose weight in the process, but it's not the focus.

You have to like what you eat. This is not an exercise in deprivation, but it's also not a free-for-all. We will focus on foods that, in addition to tasting good, make you feel good, too.

Release yourself from feelings of shame and guilt associated with food. You cannot change what you are not aware of. Instead of kicking yourself for decisions that didn't feel good, think of it as an opportunity to learn and set yourself up for success the next time you're in a similar situation.

Commit to the process. If you want to make change, you have to give it a fighting chance. New habits can take as long as six months to form. If you need accountability, I recommend getting a friend to do it with you or keeping a journal. Trust that deep down you know what's best for you. Because you do!

The Path to Food Freedom (How to Use This Book)

The first part of this book details everything you need to know about doing The Reset and achieving food freedom, including a meal-prep guide and sample Reset menus. Next come the recipes, followed by a glossary of my favorite products and resources.

The recipes, some of which are not a part of the initial Reset, are meant to be a celebration of food; easy for quick and healthy weekday meals but exciting enough to serve to your favorite friends or family members. My hope is that you'll love these recipes, and that they will spark a new way of eating. When you eat delicious, healthy foods at home, there's no need to worry about one-off or special occasions. So, order the pasta at your favorite Italian restaurant, get ice cream with your family, and enjoy your vacations. Life is too short to be stressed or to feel guilty about your food choices.

Okay, let's get started!

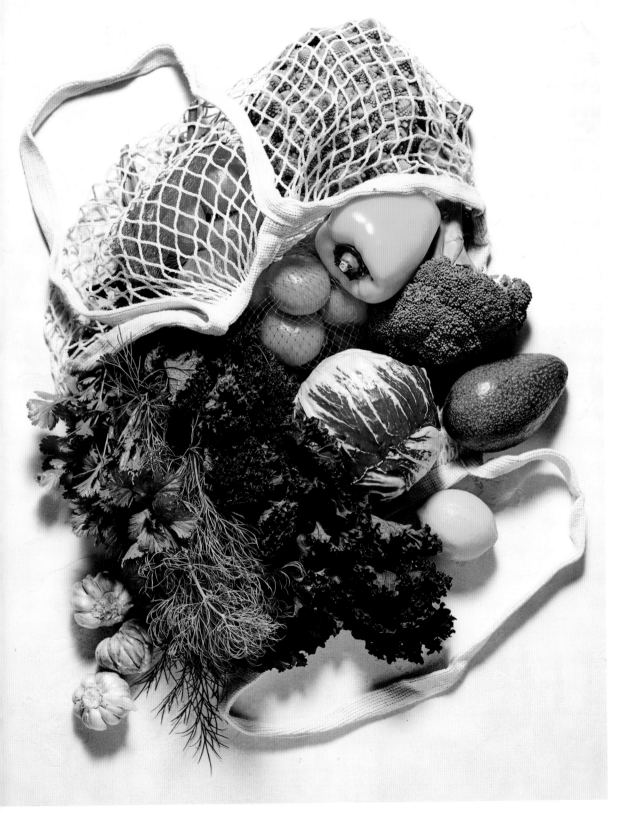

PART 1

THE PATH TO FOOD FREEDOM

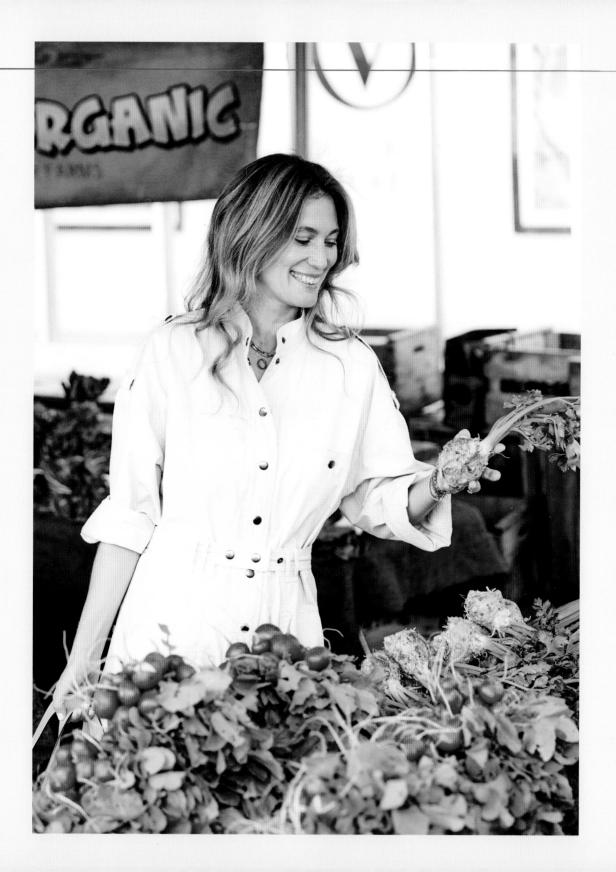

CHAPTER 1

Your Happiest, Healthiest Self Is Already in You!

If you picked up this book, I'm going to assume two things: You love food, and you want to feel good eating it.

It sounds so basic, yet for some reason, this fundamental thing that all living beings have in common has gotten so confusing.

We live in a world where it's hard to be healthy. Fast and processed foods are just too convenient, and preparing all your own meals can be a real undertaking, even for a trained chef. I have proudly become what I like to call a "one-handed cook." I want my food to taste good and feel exciting, but I, like so many others, don't have the bandwidth to cook elaborate meals each day; I need quick, easy, and flavorful options to make it work.

Trust me, I get it. For the better part of a decade, I was in constant pursuit of losing ten pounds. I felt tired and anxious all the time, my skin blemished and my clothes too tight; I needed a coffee first thing in the morning and couldn't wait for a glass of wine at the end of it; I punished myself with regular juice cleanses to make up for the fun I had over the weekend; I rarely missed a day at the gym, but the results didn't match my effort. Many of my friends seemed stuck in the same cycle. I thought it was normal to feel this way and began to accept what I felt was a fact: I would always have a little belly pooch, one or two zits, and persistent, nagging anxiety. This is who I was, and there was little I could do to change it. Well, I was dead wrong. I can honestly tell you that today I feel comfortable and confident in my body, energized, and excited about food. I eat what I want when I want, and I can't remember the last time I did a juice cleanse.

For me to break out of this slump, I had to do a few things. First and foremost, I needed to understand more about what was in the food I was eating and how it affected my physical and mental health. Starting my nutrition education was the catalyst for this shift; my relationship with food changed from restriction to abundance. I stopped yo-yo dieting and started to integrate nutrition into my everyday life. Instead of focusing on what I shouldn't have, I was intent on getting more diversity of micro- and macronutrients in every meal. As my eating patterns got more consistent, I noticed a physical and mental change, too. Physically, I could tell that my skin was brighter, clearer, and had more of a glow. My clothes definitely fit better. I felt healthy and strong, which seemed to appease the unrealistic expectations I once had for my body.

> 66 **I want my food to taste good and feel exciting, but I, like so many others, don't have the bandwidth to cook elaborate meals each day; I need quick, easy, and flavorful options to make it work.** 99

Mentally, I was more confident, happier, and less anxious. And when it came to food, this crazy thing happened: My preferences changed. I was no longer at war with my taste buds, battling between what I really wanted to eat and the "healthy" option. I genuinely enjoyed nutritious foods because I liked how they made me feel, but I wasn't fanatical about it. I could eat a French fry without spiraling into a fried food frenzy or get pizza with friends without feeling guilty, or like I "fell off the wagon." Ironically, the more I learned about nutrition, the less rigid I became and the healthier I felt. It was, and still is, absolutely liberating.

I developed The Reset as a tool to help others learn to fuel their bodies while discovering new foods and routines they truly enjoy and can easily incorporate into their daily routines. The Reset combines practical nutrition science with delicious recipes and actionable lifestyle tips to help you reach your goals and feel confident, energized, and excited about your food choices. It gives you boundaries and a plan to follow so you can break old habits that might not be serving you, while working through food dependencies and reactions to find nutrient-dense foods you actually enjoy. Results come from consistency, not extremes, and this program will help you figure out how to eat consistently in tune with your body's needs. The end goal is an effortlessly healthy lifestyle that is more fun and fulfilling than what you experienced before.

I see transformations like mine all the time—clients who come to me feeling lost and frustrated finally getting tangible results they can maintain and feel excited about. One client, a perimenopausal woman in her early fifties, came to me because she couldn't lose any weight and suffered from fatigue. Her doctor recommended hormone therapy, but she wanted to try something natural before she went that route. Three weeks and one Reset later, she lost eight pounds, and her energy levels massively increased. She never went on the hormones and was able to stay consistent with her healthy eating patterns by gaining a deeper understanding of her nutritional needs and finding new foods and routines that she genuinely enjoyed.

Another client, a forty-something male with two kids and a demanding job as a lawyer, got a wake-up call from his doctor when he found out he was thirty pounds overweight and had high cholesterol. Daily trips to Starbucks and Subway, along with a soda habit, had slowly caught up to him, and he worried about his long-term health. In just a few sessions together, we were able to find healthier alternatives to his go-to meals; we swapped a pastry for a smoothie from a local juice bar, found a salad shop that delivered, and stocked his office with healthy snacks and sugar-free soda alternatives. After making these simple changes to his everyday routine, he started to lose weight and was able to keep it off. Understanding how his food choices affected his health spurred an unexpected change; in addition to losing weight and lowering his cholesterol, his energy increased, his workouts improved, and he discovered a whole new category of foods he loved.

I always tell my clients that you don't know what it feels like to feel good until you feel *really* good. To wake up with energy and vigor, to not feel bloated, sluggish, irritable, uncomfortable in your clothes, or disappointed by your food choices—this is your natural state, we just have to find it. If I can find it, and if so many of my clients can find it, you can, too.

CHAPTER 2

Changing Your Relationship with Food

Cultivating a positive relationship with food is paramount to long-term success.

When we try to reach our goals by restricting, avoiding, and limiting our food intake, we inevitably develop an adversarial, less-is-more relationship with food. As a result, I find people end up eating similar foods each day and not feeling overly satisfied by them—think egg whites for breakfast, the same salad for lunch, a diet soda, and perhaps some plain chicken and broccoli for dinner. This might seem "safe," but it is not the most nutritious or sustainable way to eat, nor is it that enjoyable. Diet culture teaches us that we have to quantify and control our food. This is a very reductionist approach, breaking down what we eat into a static set of numbers, grading them, counting them, and placing our food choices in one of two buckets: "good" or "bad." This mindset doesn't adequately account for quality, nutrition, or the logistics of your life (i.e., schedule, who you eat with, dining out, travel, etc.). On top of all that, it's challenging to navigate all the nutrition information out there, much of which is conflicting. I feel stressed just writing about this, let alone trying to eat this way!

Instead, we're going to focus on adopting an abundance mindset toward food. Fostering curiosity and passion about ingredients, flavors, dishes, and meals makes healthy eating exciting and dynamic. We thrive when we consume a wide range of foods, which offer a variety of micro- and macronutrients. Focusing on nutrient-dense foods also leaves less room on your plate for nutrient-poor foods, like refined carbohydrates, processed foods, and sugar, without having to restrict them overtly.

Let's talk about the difference between *nutrient density* and *energy density*. I will be referring to these two terms throughout this book, so I want to make sure you clearly understand them. Nutrient density refers to the amount of nutrition (i.e., protein, fats, fiber, vitamins, minerals, phytonutrients, etc.) per serving, while energy density is a measure of calories per serving that doesn't take nutrition into account. Thanks to its high sugar content, a regular soda, for example, is very energy-dense, offering lots of calories and little nutrition per serving, while broccoli is a nutrient-dense food with a high concentration of vitamins, minerals, and other nutrients.

If you're thinking, *But I just have a sweet tooth*, you're not wrong. We are inherently pleasure seekers. Our bodies were engineered to enjoy food as a way to sustain life. This is fundamental to the human experience, and it works both for and against us. On the one hand, flavor is information; it is vitamins, minerals, phytonutrients, enzymes, and energy. On the other, our biology predisposes us to gravitate toward energy-rich foods (think sugar, carbohydrates, and fat) regardless of their nutrient density. We literally get a rush of serotonin every time we consume high-energy foods like sugar and carbohydrates. This is why we all—and yes, all of us—like pizza, pasta, cake, cookies, and bread. During times of feast and famine, this carnal desire encouraged us to stock up on energy while it was available. But evolution has not caught up with technology, and for many of us, food is now in abundance while nutrition is sadly becoming more and more scarce.

Fast-food chains and processed food companies exploit our innate desire for sustenance and pleasure with energy-rich, nutrient-poor foods that are cheap, convenient, and highly palatable. And to make things even more challenging, when we're feeling down, we crave—you guessed it—sugar! Have you ever seen a breakup movie without a heartbroken protagonist on the couch with a pint of ice cream? It's part of our nature to placate our emotions with food. And while it may feel good at the time, this momentary pleasure does not lead to long-term happiness and can actually be detrimental to your physical and mental health.

Malnutrition, which was traditionally thought of in relation to food scarcity, is now correlated with obesity because of the lack of nutrients in many foods available to us.[1] In my practice, I see laboratory results all the time from clients who have deficiencies of magnesium, B vitamins, omega-3 fatty acids, antioxidants, and other critical nutrients. We all need to eat more nutrient-dense foods while creating an environment where we can digest and absorb their nutrients. We're going to go deep into food quality and creating balanced meals later on in this book, but in a nutshell, when you consume a meal with adequate protein, fiber, and fat, you should feel more satisfied. If you find that you are consistently hungry within an hour or so of your last meal, that's a good indicator that your meal didn't have enough nutrition, your blood sugar levels are out of balance, or you're stressed, bored, or experiencing an emotional urge to eat.

Maybe in a thousand years, our body's pleasure/reward mechanism will have caught up with our modern nutrition requirements, but for now, we need to be smart about our impulses and use what we know from nutrition science along with more self-awareness and mindful eating practices to align our cravings with what our bodies need. In the moment, eating, despite the serotonin surge, does not lead to long-term happiness. In fact, study after study connects a Western diet with anxiety and depression.[2]

By contrast, traditional diets, like a Japanese or Mediterranean diet, have been linked to a 25 to 35 percent reduction in the risk for depression.[3] These traditional diets are generally based on whole, unprocessed, and home-cooked foods, while a Western diet is typically high in ultra-processed and fast foods that disrupt our blood sugar levels, nutrient intake, gut health, and essential fatty acid balance. All of which affect our mental and physical health.

The ideal ratio of omega-6 to omega-3 fatty acids, for example, is 1:1 or as high as 4:1, but the Standard American Diet (SAD) is full of processed foods and industrialized meat products that are high in omega-6 and low in omega-3 fatty acids, resulting in the consumption of twenty to thirty times more omega-6 than omega-3 fatty acids. This is not only highly inflammatory, but omega-3 fatty acid deficiencies are directly linked to an increased risk of anxiety and depression.[4] So while these processed foods have been engineered to taste amazing and feel good in the moment, we will feel happier overall when we consistently choose more nutrient-dense foods.

The magic happens when we align our food choices with our nutrient requirements. But let me calm the skeptic in you—this is not actually magic; it's science. Hormones, gut bacteria, blood sugar levels, inflammation, and many more internal and external factors contribute to how we look and feel and the foods we crave. The trick is to connect the dots between what you eat and how it makes you feel, not just in the moment you're eating, but in the hours and days that follow. Creating new associations with foods that are more dynamic than just a measure of taste makes it easier to choose the foods your body needs to thrive.

Find Your Productive Foods

By following the principles in the book, you're going to find foods that taste good, look good, smell good, and make you *feel* good; these are what I like to call *productive foods*. We each have distinct preferences, backgrounds, and physiologies, so these foods are going to be different for everyone. This is a path toward intuitive eating and food freedom. An important part of learning to eat intuitively is understanding your relationship to food and how specific foods affect your body, both positively and negatively.

When you become less reliant on substances—like sugar, refined carbohydrates, caffeine, and alcohol—and more connected to the nutritional needs of your body, you might be surprised by how effortlessly your preferences change. Breaking a sugar habit, for example, can be difficult at first, but when you get on the other end of it, you'll naturally start to crave less sugar, which can reduce anxiety, curb cravings, increase energy levels, and improve the quality of your sleep, which then helps you to be less reliant on sugar for that energy boost. As this momentum builds, continuing these healthier practices becomes easier and more enjoyable because you are in tune with your body's needs without being influenced by nutritional imbalances and food dependencies.

You cannot change what you're not aware of, so by bringing awareness to your routines, food choices, and how they make you feel, you can make informed decisions about what you want to eat and foster a more positive and productive relationship with food; it's a mindfulness practice. This is not meant to make you feel bad or shameful about yourself or something you ate, but rather to draw attention to routines and foods that might not be serving you, then help you find solutions and alternatives to improve your health and quality of life. If you eat something that doesn't feel good, but you reflect on it and learn from it, that's a win in my book. Remember, we're constantly taking a few steps forward, then a couple steps back, as we navigate our ever-changing bodies, routines, and lifestyle choices. The true transformation is in the process, not the destination.

When choosing productive foods, your enjoyment of the food is equally, if not more, important than its nutrient quality. In order to tick all the boxes, the food needs to appeal both to your senses and your physiology. For example, a hot fudge sundae might look, smell, and taste good, but it may leave you feeling a little icky. That is not a productive food, as it offers little nutrition and doesn't make you feel good. I'm not saying you should never have a hot fudge sundae, but it's not an everyday food. On the other hand, a bowl of raw vegetables sounds healthy, but might not taste great to you or it may make you bloated. This would also not be a productive food under these circumstances. As you navigate the recipes in this book, take note of the meals that feel particularly satisfying to you; perhaps you discover some well-balanced, protein-rich smoothies you enjoy, or some quick meal-prep recipes to help you make nourishing and delicious salads and bowls in a flash—now you're starting to identify productive foods that nourish your body and your taste buds.

Each of us will have our own list of productive foods, which vary based on our bodies and preferences, and once you identify one meal that ticks all your boxes, it gets easier to find more. One of my favorite recipes in the book is the Spiced Tomato and Shrimp Bisque (see page 168). I love serving this at a dinner party, as it's easy to make ahead of time (it takes only thirty minutes to prep) and is always impressive. It hits the spot for me; I love the flavor profile of spices—cumin, coriander, and turmeric—paired with succulent shrimp, grounding brown rice, and fresh herbs. I crave this dish because it's delicious and I feel great after eating it. As you navigate through The Reset and this book, take note of the productive foods you discover. Make a list, and continue adding to it until you have an arsenal of productive foods available to you. They can include recipes, meal-prep favorites, frozen foods, takeout, and dishes from your favorite restaurants.

A New Paradigm
The Four Pillars of Health

The more I learn about the human body, the more awestruck I am by it. I firmly believe that the body's natural state is health. We were engineered to heal ourselves. Isn't it amazing how you can cut your finger and new skin forms around it? That when you get an infection, you develop a fever to kill the virus or bacteria that caused it? And, if you've ever followed the field of epigenetics, how wild is it that your behavior and choices can change the way your genes are expressed? We are living, breathing, and constantly evolving beings, and our bodies are continuously replacing damaged cells and tissue with healthy new ones.

So, what does it mean to truly be *healthy*? Health is not merely the absence of illness or disease, but rather a state of physical, mental, social, and spiritual well-being that allows you to function optimally and offers resilience against illness or injury.[5] Take two people, both with a broken leg; one person exercises regularly, eats a whole foods diet, and has minimal stress; the other leads a sedentary lifestyle, eats a diet mainly of processed and fast food, and has a lot of stress. Who do you think is going to be more resilient and heal faster?

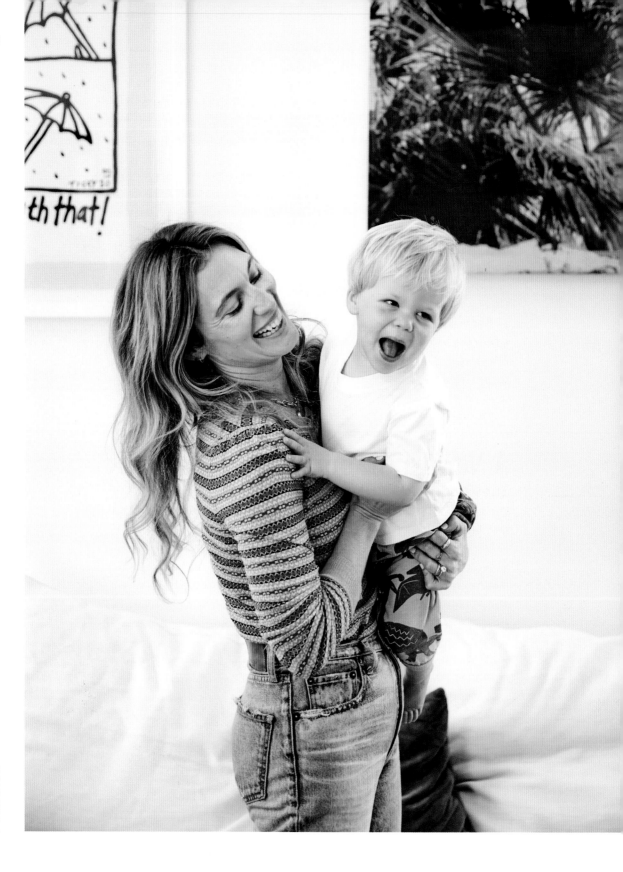

The Four Pillars of Health

Physical:	**Mental:**	**Social:**	**Spiritual:**
Nutrition, Strength, Endurance	Awareness, Decision-Making, Focus, Attitude	Family, Community	Morals, Core Values, Purpose

When I say that your happiest, healthiest self is already in you, I am talking about nourishing all four of these pillars because your health is more complex than counting calories or avoiding dairy; it's not about weight, muscle tone, or the firmness of your skin, it's about finding that sweet spot where you feel supported mentally, physically, socially, and spiritually.

It's a delicate dance to keep these four pillars in balance. If you prioritize your physical health so much that you feel stressed or anxious about going out for dinner with friends or family, that might negatively affect your mental and social health. Or, if you're out every night indulging in food and wine, your social pillar might be overflowing at the detriment of your physical and mental health, and perhaps even compromising some of your values.

Community and family are incredibly important, and food can often be an immense form of comfort that we reach for to enhance or supplement social connection. We cannot prioritize our nutrition at the expense of this connection, disregard the impact of food (both positive and negative) on our mental health, or put our morals and values on the back burner. There is a stark difference between eating a packaged cookie alone in your car after a stressful day at work and eating one of your grandmother's famous holiday cookies at a family gathering, even if they have the same nutrition profile. The latter might conjure joyous memories of your childhood, is shared with loved ones, and feels celebratory. While the cookie may be nutrient-poor on paper, eating it is a soul-nourishing activity. Now, I wouldn't recommend eating a dozen of them or having them every day, but the point I'm trying to make is that nutrition isn't binary; foods aren't either "good" or "bad," and true health is much more than what we eat.

Our unrelenting diet culture can turn otherwise happy indulgences into a spiral of shame or a cascade of self-sabotaging choices. It's too easy to get evangelical about health foods and nutrition ideology, while turning a blind eye to other choices we make that are not supportive of our overall health. In *Foodwise*, we are focusing on the big picture of your health, flexibility over rigidity, and having a greater understanding of your physical and emotional needs so you can be effortlessly more consistent, eat in harmony with how you live, and ultimately have greater health outcomes.

Diets Don't Work, but This Does

You should eat what makes you feel good, and how you eat should be a part of how you live. Full stop. Trying to look, eat, or behave like someone else is not only wholly unrealistic but also maddening. For those of you searching for the holy grail, I'm going to tell you straight: There is no such thing as the perfect body or diet; instead, each of us has a way of eating and living that will feel right. We just have to find it somewhere beneath the layers of misinformation, confusion, unfair societal pressures, and negative self-talk.

Our broken diet culture has taken enjoyment away from eating and replaced it with stress, fear, and utter confusion about what and how to eat. We are bombarded with conflicting information about what's good and what's bad for us, and the promises of quick fixes are just as tempting as they are bewildering. The noise has become so loud that it's drowned out our inner voice and intuition, leaving us tired, sick, and constantly searching for the next trend that will make us well. This, combined with the collective stress of the modern world, and ultra-processed and fast foods, makes change hard to come by.

It's widely accepted that the way to lose weight is to "eat less, move more." If you ask me, that's just a recipe for hunger, and research shows that most dieters end up gaining all the weight back (and often more!). Here are some of the ways The Reset trains you for success:

Focus on taste and abundance over restriction: The Reset uses an easy-to-follow meal plan that emphasizes enjoyment, satisfaction, and the discovery of productive foods that taste as good as they make you feel. So much of the dieting information we get is too restrictive to fit into everyday life, ultimately setting us up to fail. The Reset boils it down to the lowest common denominators—gluten, dairy, sugar, processed food, alcohol, and coffee. The idea is not to avoid these foods forever, but rather to help you evaluate your relationship with them, while offering a plethora of delicious alternatives so you never feel deprived.

Crafted around long-term solutions: The goal of The Reset is to establish routines that support your body and can be realistically continued long after the program is complete. This is not a quick fix, but rather a jump start. By exploring new foods and uncovering foods that don't serve you well, you can create new habits that are enjoyable, supportive of your goals, and (most important) doable.

Create a personalized plan: There is no one-size-fits-all meal plan. During the twenty-one-day Reset, you will do the work to find foods and lifestyle solutions that suit your preferences, physiology, and the way you live your life. With this information, you can feel more confident in your food choices as they pertain specifically to *you*. The Reset also offers a lot of flexibility if you need to adjust the plan during the program.

The food actually tastes good: On The Reset, every day is an opportunity to try something new that you love. There are plenty of Reset-friendly recipes in this book for you to try, but you are not limited to them. I encourage you get creative, try new things, or tweak your favorite meals to make them more productive. The intersection of nutrition and pleasure is your sweet spot. When you love your healthy foods, it's easy to be consistent, and that is when you get real results.

Nourish mind, body, and soul simultaneously: The Reset is not simply a meal plan; the goal is to find a way of eating and living that supports better sleep, reduced stress, and feeling more energetic, motivated, and productive so you can be the best version of you. Food is an important element to this, and through this program, you will understand how to nourish with and beyond food. Through this program you will learn how to set yourself up for success and promote optimal health by nourishing yourself with and beyond food.

Success is a feeling, not a number: When you shift the focus away from weight and toward energy, mood, sleep, stress reduction, and overall health, you might be surprised that you feel more comfortable in your skin without having to put so much pressure on the scale. I've had many clients over the years come to me with a specific number in mind that they'd like to weigh; interestingly, they get partly there, feel great, and no longer care about that number.

You are the expert of your body, and if something doesn't feel right, it probably isn't. In my nutrition practice, I like to blend the clinical with the practical, or the qualitative with the quantitative. It's easy to brush symptoms—such as fatigue, stomach ailments, stress, weight fluctuations, skin rashes, and blemishes—aside, but these all can be treated and improved with nutrition and lifestyle changes. The challenge is finding new routines that you can and want to keep up. Being overly ambitious about dietary or lifestyle changes backfires more often than not. The Reset is an opportunity to find new wellness practices that you are excited to continue because you enjoy them, and love the way they make you feel. Here are a few important points to consider when thinking about the best foods and routines for you:

Convenience. I operate off of a "good, better, best" mentality. While I love the idea of cooking and meal prepping, for most of us (myself included!), cooking all our meals at home is not realistic. Try a blend of home-cooked meals, easy-to-assemble meals, frozen meals, and prepared meals (including takeout!) so you always have a healthy option available for you. Make a plan, test it, then tweak it until you have a delicious, healthy, and accessible food list. I have a list of premade food brands in the Resources section to get you started, and I recommend that you keep some more convenient options on your list of productive foods.

Pleasure. You have to like the food if you are going to continue eating it. Think about what foods do you like and what don't you like. Do you prefer warm over cold foods? Do you absolutely hate kale, cilantro, or eggplant? Do you like to cook, and if so, how much time do you realistically have for it? Do you need to plan ahead so you can eat at regular times and truly enjoy your meals?

I have so many clients who don't want to make smoothies because they don't want to clean the blender. This might sound silly, but it's a legitimate reason why some people don't make smoothies for breakfast. Acknowledge your roadblocks and find realistic alternatives or solutions. For this one, I would recommend a personal blender, so you don't have to wash it out immediately (check the Resources section for specific brands I recommend).

Accessibility. Do you have an erratic work schedule, family members with specific food preferences, or dietary restrictions? Are you in school and struggling to find healthy on-campus options, or do you live and eat with picky eaters who are not open to new foods? Think about your life, schedule, culture, family traditions, and more, and make sure to account for these. It might require a little strategic thinking or trial and error, but there is always a workaround.

Consistency. What you do most of the time matters more than what you do some of the time. Make sure you are setting yourself up for success. Think about where you will be at mealtimes and have a plan in place. Are you starving every day at four p.m. and don't have a healthy snack option? Do you get home from work famished and snack your way until dinner? Or do you limit your food intake early in the day, only to find yourself overdoing it in the evening? It's critical that you enjoy and are satisfied by your healthy meals so you will feel motivated to continue eating them. Find easy breakfasts, lunches, dinners, and snacks that you like and can eat regularly, and enjoy special occasions and meals thoroughly and guilt-free.

Your body is giving you clues all day, every day, about what it needs to be nourished. You just need to find that awareness so you can react to these clues. Whether you're struggling with energy levels, weight, digestion, mood, skin problems, hormonal fluctuations, stress, poor sleep, an autoimmune condition, or gut dysbiosis, I am here to tell you that you can make a positive change all on your own, and it only takes twenty-one days to get started.

It's time to get in the driver's seat. Instead of a one-size-fits-all, short-term meal plan, what you'll get from this book is a path toward breaking food dependencies, learning about your body, and finding real foods that you actually like eating, which will help you achieve your goals, and make you feel great.

PART 2

THE RESET

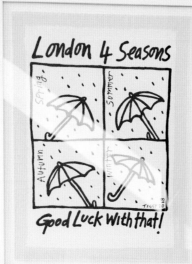

London 4 Seasons

Spring Summer

Autumn Winter

Good Luck With that!

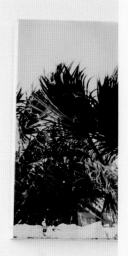

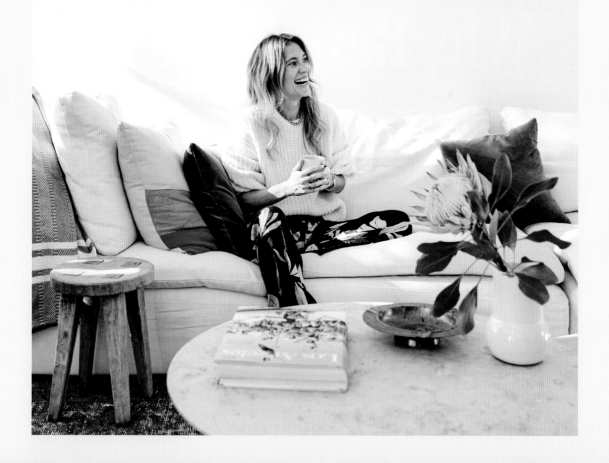

CHAPTER 3

Why Reset?

Many people underestimate how amazing it feels to wake up rested, clear-minded, and ready for the day; not be dependent on sugar, coffee, or alcohol to get started or wind down; feel comfortable in your clothes and confident in your skin.

Our lives are so nonstop, we might not even realize how much better we can feel or that we have the power to change it. We all know what it feels like to be out of your groove—maybe you don't jump out of bed every morning ready to take on the day; you might lack the energy to explore your interests or the activities that make you feel good like exercising, reading, cooking, or spending quality time with your friends and family; or maybe you are irritable, bloated, or anxious and, above all, tired all the time. Sometimes you need a break to reconnect with the healthy habits you once thrived on, create new ones you can stick with, and discover what works for your body and lifestyle so you can feel your absolute best.

Detoxification and cleansing are ancient methods for ridding toxins from the body and fostering optimal health. These traditions date back centuries and have been documented in early Roman, Native American, Indian, and Chinese cultures. They're not meant to be a quick fix, but rather a jump start. I developed The Reset through years of personal experience, extensive studies, and client work. And let me tell you this: Sometimes, it's easier just to rip the Band-Aid off and have a plan to follow so we will actually do the thing. I have clients who have been dabbling for years with eating less sugar, drinking less wine, and cutting back on coffee or processed foods, but have never actually committed enough for it to make a difference and change their habits.

Needing a Reset doesn't mean you're unhealthy, unvirtuous, or need to punish yourself for living too large; it's an opportunity to take a time-out from our 24-7 lives to rest, heal, and reevaluate the choices we make with a deeper understanding of our needs. This twenty-one-day program provides a structure and boundaries for you to be introspective while giving your body meaningful time and space to rest and heal. You will work through food dependencies and possibly even identify food reactions while increasing your nutrition knowledge to find a way of eating and living uniquely suited to your body and lifestyle.

I have been doing a version of The Reset once or twice a year for a decade, and each time I am amazed by how good I feel and the new habits I develop. I like to use my semi-annual Reset to reconnect with myself and consider how my body and circumstances may have changed. Old routines are old routines. What may have worked well for you in the past might not be the best fit for your physiology and lifestyle today. It's important to be flexible with your wellness rituals and learn to listen to your body so you can adjust as necessary. We often underestimate how changes like a new job, city, or partner can disrupt your routine. Working from home or transitioning back into the office can have its challenges as well. And kids, as much as we love them, really throw a wrench into things; it's harder to cook and workout, and you

> **❝ Sometimes you need a break to reconnect with the healthy habits you once thrived on, create new ones you can stick with, and discover what works for your body and lifestyle so you can feel your absolute best. ❞**

have infinitely less time for yourself. Trying to fit your old routines into your new life is frustrating and usually unsuccessful, but The Reset is the perfect way to adjust those routines so they can work for your life as it is today.

The Reset is not a magic cure; it's a new beginning. Consider this an opportunity to reestablish your relationship with sugar, gluten, dairy, caffeine, alcohol, and other foods you may not tolerate well while discovering new productive foods and routines that align with your body's needs and the demands of your lifestyle. Food influences so much more than just weight; it can impact how we sleep, our stress levels, mood, energy levels, and ultimately our resilience to illness and injury. Whether you've experienced a significant life change like marriage, a move, new job, or baby, or simply feel a little "off" or out of your groove, The Reset is a great way to jump-start food and lifestyle routines that will help you thrive in all areas of your life.

You should approach any nutrition program as an educational experience. There is a lot of information out there, and I hope that by reading this book and following the principles I've laid out here, you will have a deeper understanding not only of your body but also the field of nutrition in general. There are many different methods and theories, and I'm honored that you're reading this book to hear mine. I like to equate seeking nutrition advice to seeking parenting advice. When I was expecting my son, Ozzie, I was given a lot of "tips." I immediately forgot most of them, but this stuck with me: If you ask five different people for parenting advice, you will get five different answers—choose one person you trust and whose approach you like to ask all your questions. Your health is pretty similar: Choose a nutrition approach that speaks to you and stay consistent with it. Doing a little of a lot of different things isn't going to get you the results you want and will most likely just confuse you in the process.

The true value of The Reset isn't in the twenty-one days you're doing it, but in how you apply what you learn to your everyday post-Reset life. The goal is to feel confident in your food and lifestyle choices and get into a rhythm where eating a nutrient-rich diet is effortless, enjoyable, and intuitive. This is when the frustrating and futile cycle of trying fad diet after fad diet ends, and you just start living.

You will see many recurring themes and topics in the information that follows. There's a lot of overlap between sleep, stress, hormone fluctuations, digestion, immune function, reproduction, skin health, and everything else your body does. This is not meant to be repetitive but to show how connected the systems of the body are.

If you took the shift key off your computer's keyboard, for example, it would affect a lot more than the keyboard's appearance. You wouldn't be able to capitalize letters; make an exclamation point, dollar sign, or asterisk; and you wouldn't be able to take a screenshot using the keyboard. It would affect word processing, emailing, and typing passwords, along with probably everything else you do on your computer. It's the same in our bodies: When one key is missing, it affects the whole system. So, let's adopt a more integrated view. If you get a headache or a zit, think beyond the superficial to treat it and prevent it from coming back. And if it keeps happening, dig deeper!

Some of this might feel science-heavy, but I want you to understand the *why* and think about how it might relate to your body and life. Use this information to connect the dots between any symptoms you might be experiencing and the underlying cause, and to monitor any changes. The more you know about what is happening internally, the better The Reset will resonate.

Understanding Food Reactions

The first step in figuring out your relationship with and tolerance level of specific foods is understanding the differences between the three types of food reactions: allergies, sensitivities, and intolerances. We often accept our fatigue, digestive issues, headaches, weight gain, lack of energy, brain fog, mood swings, anxiety, skin problems, joint pain, or poor sleep as part of us, but sometimes simply removing a specific food can vastly improve or eliminate these symptoms. You don't need to be eating unhealthy foods to have a food reaction. As you'll learn, sometimes a perfectly healthy food might not be the right food for you, or a food you once avoided might not be that bad for you after all. The Reset will help you gain clarity over any food reactions you may have while giving your immune and digestive systems a break, and your gut a chance to heal.

Food reactions are complex and, in my opinion, often misunderstood and oversimplified. One of the most profound benefits of doing The Reset is discovering your tolerance level to specific foods and adjusting your relationship with those foods accordingly. Now, this doesn't mean necessarily eliminating more foods from your diet. You very well may discover that a particular food—take gluten or dairy, for example— really doesn't make you feel good and decide you want to avoid it moving forward. You could also find out that certain amounts of gluten and dairy in some forms are okay for you, so you can confidently enjoy it. Food reactions are not always black and white; you may have some level of tolerance of foods people are commonly sensitive to, meaning you can eat specific amounts or certain types of this food without it negatively affecting your health. I like to think of it as a spectrum with lots of shades of grey.

Food Allergies

You probably already know if you have a food allergy, as it can be dangerous and even life-threatening. The most common food allergens are cow's milk, eggs, peanuts, tree nuts, soy, wheat, whitefish, and shellfish. These true allergies are diagnosed through a blood test showing IgE antibodies. Antibodies are proteins found in the blood that serve as the memory of the immune system. When you have IgE antibodies to a specific food and consume it, your immune system starts to attack it. The symptoms often present themselves within a few minutes to a few hours and can include the closing of the throat, wheezing, coughing, diarrhea, vomiting, hives, an itchy rash, or swelling in the face, mouth, or tongue. In The Reset, we are not looking for food allergies because I am assuming that you already know if you have one, and I don't want to unnecessarily eliminate otherwise healthy foods, like nuts and seafood, if you are not allergic to them. If you have even mild forms of the aforementioned symptoms, I'd recommend consulting an allergist to get tested.

Food Sensitivities

Like allergies, food sensitivities also elicit an immune response, characterized by IgG and IgA antibodies triggered by food, chemicals, or bacteria. They are caused by increased gut permeability, a condition also known as *leaky gut*, where food particles get into the bloodstream and trigger an immune response. Sensitivities generally involve a milder and delayed response. Symptoms can take hours or days to manifest and include headaches, fatigue, runny nose, reflux, joint pain, skin irritations (think acne, flushing, itchiness, or rashes like eczema or psoriasis), digestive issues, nausea, or brain fog. Because of this delayed response and the ways they present themselves, food sensitivities are hard to pinpoint. You might not realize that your Thursday afternoon bout of fatigue was from the pasta you ate Tuesday night, but given how food sensitivities operate, that's entirely possible. Food sensitivities are also cumulative, which means the more you eat the offending food, the stronger the reaction will be.

You can be sensitive to any type of food, but 80 percent of food sensitivities come from beef, citrus, dairy products, eggs, corn, pork, and wheat products.[6] These foods aren't *bad*, in fact they can be highly nutritious; they just might not be the right foods for some people.

Food Intolerances

A food intolerance is an issue digesting and breaking down a specific food. It could come from an enzyme deficiency, a naturally occurring chemical, or another sensitivity, and causes symptoms like bloating, nausea, gas, diarrhea, cramping, headaches, or (what I like to call) a nervous belly—you know that nagging feeling?

Lactose intolerance is the most common type of food intolerance and is caused by a deficiency in the enzyme lactase, which helps break down lactose, a sugar that is naturally found in dairy products. Lactose intolerance is separate from a cow's milk allergy or sensitivity but can be uncomfortable nonetheless. Seventy-five percent of the world's population has a lactose intolerance. It is especially prevalent in those of African, Asian, Middle Eastern, Mediterranean, and Jewish descent, but a lactose intolerance doesn't mean you have to swear off all dairy products for good. For example, I stay away from milk and cream-based foods but do well with cheese, especially sheep's and goat's milk products. This is probably because fermented forms of dairy like cheese, cultured butter, and yogurt have less lactose, if any at all. In the fermentation process, the yeast eats away at the carbohydrate (in this case, lactose), so the longer the fermentation, the less lactose there is. Also, sheep's and goat's milks are naturally lower in lactose than cow's, so that could be a good option for you, depending on your tolerance level. If your issue with dairy is really with the lactose, these might be options to explore during the reintroduction phase so you're not stuck with a cheese-less life.

Gluten sensitivities aren't cut-and-dried, either. Celiac disease, which we hear a lot about these days, is an autoimmune condition triggered by gluten consumption and doesn't fall into these food reaction categories. Approximately 1 in 100 people, or 1 percent of the population, has celiac. But celiac aside, you can have an allergy, intolerance, or sensitivity to gluten or wheat, the primary gluten source.

Quick-cooking techniques, often used for making bread, pasta, and other gluten-containing products, don't allow the gluten to thoroughly cook, making it more difficult to digest. Fermenting and sprouting wheat products makes them a lot easier on the stomach. In fact, fermented gluten products like sourdough bread have less gluten in them. In the fermentation process (similar to the dairy example above), bacteria break down carbohydrates and gluten, making the end product easier to digest and increasing nutrient absorption. Most wheat available in the United States is also sprayed with pesticides, which can cause a reaction independent of gluten. If you eat gluten, you might feel better with organic, non-GMO wheat products, which generally aren't sprayed with as many pesticides.

These aren't solutions for everyone, especially those with celiac, but through this process, you will figure out what your tolerance level of gluten is—it doesn't have to be all or nothing. By choosing the right products and eating them in the right frequency (i.e., not every day or maybe even not every week), you may still be able to enjoy some of your favorite gluten-containing foods, even if you have a reaction to them.

An elimination diet—where you remove a food for a period of time, then reintroduce it to gauge the reaction—is the gold standard for discovering food sensitivities and intolerances. That is what we will be doing on The Reset. The ultimate goal is to safely and confidently enjoy as many foods as possible, and after completing this program, you will know how a particular food affects you once and for all.

When it comes to food sensitivities and intolerances, in particular, a strong and healthy gut can open up more foods for you. Part of the value in The Reset is creating an environment to digest foods more efficiently and absorb more nutrients. Understanding how you react to specific foods also gives you more control over any symptoms that might be frustrating you. Perhaps gluten makes you feel a little bloated, but it's pizza night with your best friends. Pizza might not be an everyday food for you, but you get to make that cost-benefit analysis, knowing how the food will make you feel.

The Limitations of Testing

Understanding the connection between what you eat and how you feel is one way The Reset can be game-changing. It's tempting to want to just take a test, and while food reactivity testing is improving, there are some inherent flaws.

- Most of these tests are for food sensitivities only. They are looking specifically for IgG and IgA immune responses, which (as we now know) are not the only indicators of a food reaction.

- There is no standard for non-IgE (true allergy) antibody testing, which means that you will probably get different results depending on the test you take.

- You have to be eating the foods you are sensitive to for it to show a reaction in the test.

- If you have a leaky gut, foods you commonly eat might show up in your results, which doesn't necessarily mean that you're sensitive to that food. Many clients come to me freaked out about being sensitive to foods they eat regularly, but these results can be misleading. When I see a test with many food sensitivities, I focus on gut healing over permanently removing these foods.

- Most people produce IgG antibodies after eating food, so the presence of these antibodies might not be a sensitivity at all but a typical response from exposure to that food.

- Food sensitivities are not a forever diagnosis. They can often be corrected through gut healing, so avoiding specific foods permanently after a single test is not an appropriate treatment approach and may lead to nutrient deficiencies and overly restrictive eating patterns.

Weight Loss

While most people who want to lose weight on this program will, I want you to use this time to shift your focus away from the number on the scale and toward your physical and mental well-being. When you align these forces, your weight will settle at a healthy place for you and your body. If you are stepping on the scale, make sure to give yourself a three- to five-pound goal weight range, rather than just a fixed number. Our weight is not static, and there are many factors beyond adipose tissue (fat) that contribute to that number. Make sure you are also considering other metrics for progress alongside weight, including how your clothes fit, your energy levels, mood, skin, and the quality of your sleep. The number on the scale is not the end all be all. Taking the pressure and the mind games out of trying to land on one ideal number is absolutely liberating and can be supportive of the other benefits of The Reset, especially reduced stress.

Reduce Stress

Stress lives in many forms, but we often pay the most attention to emotional stress; this is when you feel "stressed out" about work, being stuck in traffic, or having an argument with a loved one. Other forms of stress include physical stress, which can come from pain, excessive exercise, illness or injury, environmental stress from toxins, alcohol, sugar, allergens, or extreme temperatures; and inherited stress, which can come from genetics, pregnancy, and other factors that are mostly out of your hands. The cumulative burden of stress on your body is your *allostatic load*. And while we may not eradicate all stress during The Reset, we can reduce your overall stress levels by removing some food and lifestyle triggers. Think of your allostatic load like a backpack filled with a book for each stressor. The fewer stressors you have, the easier it is for your body to handle. Too many stressors can create a burden you're not able to shoulder, and lead to burnout.

To fully grasp the impact of stress, it's important to understand the science behind this reaction. *Cortisol*, our primary stress hormone, is made by the adrenal glands and regulated by the *HPA axis*, which connects our adrenal glands (which sit above the kidneys) to the hypothalamus and pituitary gland in our brain. When we experience a stressful event, whether environmental, physical, or emotional, our HPA axis directs the adrenals to increase stress hormone output, which elevates blood glucose levels and stimulates the fight-or-flight response. In fight-or-flight, the sympathetic nervous system (SNS) is activated and the body turns off functions that aren't helpful in an immediate life-or-death situation, like digestion, immune response, reproduction, and growth, while increasing your heart rate, blood glucose levels, and stress hormones. When the stressful event is perceived to be over, the parasympathetic nervous system (PNS) is activated, which is often referred to as the "rest and digest" system, and relaxes the body.

Since the effects of stress are cumulative, when we experience chronic (long-term) stress, we build resistance to cortisol fluctuations, making it more difficult for the HPA axis to bring the body back to normal levels. Nonessential bodily functions are also impaired; the immune system might be working at a lower capacity, leaving us vulnerable to illness and inflammation; digestion can slow down, leading to bacterial overgrowth, bloating, nutrition imbalances, leaky gut, food sensitivities, other digestive issues, and skin issues; fertility may be affected and, in women, PMS symptoms heightened. Many of these stress-related ailments are treatable conditions on their own—we can adopt a new skincare routine for the acne or work on our sleep hygiene for better rest—but when we address the symptoms alone, we aren't solving the problem.

The good news is that you can reduce the impact of stress on your body system with dietary and lifestyle interventions that are good for you regardless of your stress levels. The Reset follows a pattern of eating that is optimal for stress management and activating the parasympathetic nervous system, which includes an abundance of leafy greens, high-quality proteins, and complex carbohydrates in the form of a balanced breakfast, hearty lunch, and a lighter, earlier dinner. These foods and activities will promote better sleep, cortisol regulation, nourishment of your adrenal glands and HPA axis, and improve your energy levels, among other stress-reducing benefits.

Heal Your Gut & Improve Digestion

The Reset is an opportunity for your gut to rest and heal, and for you to identify potential digestive triggers. The program removes common gut disruptors, like sugar, gluten, alcohol, and processed foods, while adding in therapeutic foods known to improve gut health, including probiotic-containing fermented foods, prebiotic-rich fruits and vegetables, leafy greens, collagen, and bone broth in the form of healing soups. Dietary changes, along with improved sleep and reduced stress levels, can significantly improve your gut health, digestion, and nearly every part of your body. Through the process, you will also gain a deeper understanding of the foods that nourish your body (as well as what doesn't), and how to make informed choices when your Reset is complete.

The term *gut health* specifically refers to the balance and function of bacteria present throughout the digestive tract, or alimentary canal, which begins in the mouth and goes all the way through to the rectum. Because the alimentary canal is open to the external environment at each end, our digestive system is considered "outside" of the body.

The primary functions of the gut are the digestion of food, absorption of nutrients, and excretion of waste. The gut helps us break down food into nutrients that enter the bloodstream and travel throughout the body to where they are needed. Nearly 70 percent of the immune system lies within the gut; it protects us from viruses, bacteria, or other pathogens but can also work against us when things go awry, contributing to autoimmune diseases, food allergies, or food sensitivities.

There are approximately 100 trillion bacteria in our gut, known as the microbiome. In addition to regulating digestion, the makeup of these bacteria has real health implications. Gut dysbiosis, or imbalance, causes some uncomfortable side effects, like constipation, diarrhea, heartburn, belching, and bloating, and can lead to nutrient deficiencies that affect everything from our cognitive skills and energy levels to the strength of our bones, muscle mass, and immune function. Key disruptors to gut health include stress; lack of sleep; medication use, including NSAIDs like aspirin or ibuprofen and antibiotics; and, of course, food, especially sugar, alcohol, and processed foods.

Many of our "happy hormones," including GABA, dopamine, and about 95 percent of our body's serotonin, are produced in the gut. Vitamin B6, magnesium, and the amino acid tryptophan are all essential nutrients for serotonin production, which means that we not only need to consume these nutrients but also digest and absorb them properly; we need a strong and healthy gut for this. Interestingly, people often report gastrointestinal (GI) issues alongside mental health conditions; 70 to 90 percent of people with irritable bowel syndrome (IBS) also suffer from a mood or anxiety disorder. By increasing nutrient intake and absorption, The Reset can help improve your digestive comfort, as well as your mood and mental health.

Other important functions of the gut include regulation of metabolism and the cardiovascular system (this includes cholesterol and triglyceride levels), which has enormous implications given the shocking statistic that only 12 percent of Americans are considered metabolically healthy[7]—defined as having ideal blood sugar, triglycerides, cholesterol, blood pressure, and weight levels without the use of medication. Using The Reset as a tool to jump-start healthier habits supportive of gut and overall health can be incredibly beneficial for one's general well-being and quality of life.

Balance Blood Sugar Levels

On The Reset, a focus on balanced meals with protein, fiber, and fat, along with reduced sugar and refined carbohydrate intake, will help you recalibrate your blood sugar levels for more sustained energy and fewer cravings throughout the day. To better understand this concept, let's take a look at how carbohydrates are metabolized.

Carbohydrates from grains, vegetables, and anything with sugar get broken down into glucose (or sugar) molecules. Glucose is the dominant source of ATP, or energy, and is tightly regulated by the hormones insulin and glucagon. When our blood sugar levels are too high, insulin tells our muscles, liver, and fat cells to store glucose; conversely, when our blood sugar levels are low, the hormone glucagon is released to increase our blood sugar levels.

Managing your blood sugar levels can significantly impact the quality of your life and your ability to reach your health and wellness goals. Still, it is more complex than avoiding carbohydrates altogether. By eating whole food sources of carbohydrates like whole grains, fruits, and vegetables, you will get the added benefit of fiber to help slow digestion and blood sugar peaks. This reduces the *glycemic index*, a scale that represents the amount a particular food spikes your blood sugar levels. Numbers of the glycemic index range from 1 to 100, with a higher number indicating a more significant spike. For example, white rice has a glycemic index of 72, while its whole grain counterpart, brown rice, has 50. This means you'll experience less of a spike when eating brown rice. You can also reduce blood sugar spikes by pairing a higher-GI food with protein, fiber, and fat. For example, when we eat an apple with almond butter, we will experience less of a spike than if we ate the apple alone or just drank apple juice.

Pay attention to your energy levels and cravings before and after The Reset. You may find that as your glycemic load reduces, you'll get used to eating fewer carbohydrates and feel satisfied with less. If you want to dig deeper, you can get a continuous glucose monitor to measure your blood sugar fluctuations throughout the day. I have a recommendation for this in the Resources section. It can be an interesting exercise to try for a month and learn more about how to optimize your metabolic health.

Improved Sleep

When you're constantly on the go and have a demanding job, an active social life, and/or a family, sleep can fall to the bottom of the list of priorities. Inadequate sleep, defined by length, quality, and regularity, is an all too common problem, and it doesn't just make us tired in the morning. It can trigger a cascade of physical and emotional consequences, including increased stress, memory and cognitive impairment, elevated hunger levels and sugar cravings, accelerating aging, inflammation, a weakened immune system, and more.

Food plays a significant role in the quality of your sleep. Whether you're eating poorly because you're sleeping poorly or the other way around, processed foods, sugar, overeating, excessive alcohol, and caffeine intake can impair sleep. When you eat can also affect your sleep. Our body receives cues from daylight and the timing of our meals to manage our internal clock. When this is thrown off from travel, night shift work (ahem, new parents), or erratic eating patterns, our sleep is often affected.

Reducing stress and inflammation, balancing blood sugar levels, and exercising can also support your sleep. During The Reset, you'll have the opportunity to truly rest. You may find that you're tired in the beginning—that's your body, without stimulants, telling you it's exhausted. Lean into that, give yourself some rest, and take note of how your body feels with consistently good sleep.

Conquer Food Cravings

A food craving is when you experience an intense desire to consume a specific food. Most cravings come from sugary, fatty, or salty foods. There are many reasons why we develop cravings, and I think it's safe to assume we've all experienced it at some point in our lives. However, not dissimilar to drugs or alcohol, the more we indulge in these cravings, the higher a tolerance we will have for them, meaning we will need to increase the quantity and frequency of the food we're craving to feel satisfied. Momentarily satisfied, that is. Here are a few reasons why we crave foods and how we'll handle them on The Reset.

Blood Sugar Fluctuations

High-carbohydrate meals without adequate protein, fiber, and fat can make you tired, irritable, and reaching for more foods that will increase your blood sugar levels after the initial rush subsides. Have you ever experienced an onset of hunger where your hands are almost shaking? When, despite your best intentions, you grab a bag of potato chips while waiting in line to order a salad? I like to call this *hang-ziety*, and it's often related to erratic blood sugar levels. Focusing on blood sugar regulation is critical to reducing sugar and carbohydrate cravings. This is precisely what we'll be doing on The Reset, starting with a well-balanced, protein-rich smoothie for breakfast.

Stress

Wanting to pacify our emotions with food is an experience we can all relate to. Studies show that chronic stress directly connects to food cravings and weight gain[8] by increasing our desire for foods that activate our pleasure/reward center and provide some temporary relief from the stressor. Many foods like dairy products, and wheat also contain *exorphins*, a naturally occurring proteins that act similarly to opioids to make us feel good and decrease pain. Exorphins can lead to addictive behavior, and make us crave foods that we don't tolerate well, especially when stressed.

Additionally, cravings for salty foods can indicate HPA axis dysfunction, which is estimated to affect as many as 80 percent of Americans.[9] No wonder we like chips so much!

Sleep

The quality of our sleep is deeply connected to our food cravings. At the most basic level, when you're tired, you're going to want more stimulants like caffeine, refined carbohydrates, and sugar to give you more energy. Sleep is also crucial for regulating our metabolism, and lack of sleep can lead to imbalances in leptin and ghrelin (our hunger hormones) and increased cravings as a result.

Hormonal Changes

Natural hormonal changes can lead to increased hunger, cravings, and decreased satisfaction after eating. Getting adequate nutrition, reducing stress, and sleeping better (which go hand in hand with

During the luteal phase of menstruation, estrogen is low and progesterone is high—a recipe for increased cravings. It's become a culturally accepted joke that women want chocolate during their period, but this is an actual biological event. Lean into this by eating more whole grains and quality sweets, so you can be in control of these cravings and mitigate excessive blood sugar spikes and a potential avalanche of unproductive food choices that will make you feel worse. There are some great recipes in this book (I love the Reset-friendly Salted Caramel Chocolate Fudge on page 198 and the Chocolate-Avocado Mousse on page 202), but you can also buy high-quality chocolates and other indulgences, even on The Reset.

nutrition) are vital for hormonal regulation. When you're consistent with these habits, normal fluctuations in your menstruation cycle or hormonal changes from stress or other life events (including pregnancy and menopause) may feel less dramatic, leading to fewer cravings.

Learned Habits

Cravings can be habitual, and these habits are hard to break. Always want popcorn during a movie or something sweet after dinner? Do you feel like you can't get started with your workday without a pilgrimage to the local coffee shop for a vanilla latte? These are behaviors that we have learned over time. Sometimes, going cold turkey is the best way to disrupt those types of cravings. Sure, the first couple days can be challenging, especially if this is a daily habit, but stick with it, and it will eventually lose its appeal. And remember: You eat what you see, so clean out your pantry before starting The Reset, and set yourself up with healthier alternatives to your favorite foods.

Not all cravings are bad, and as you reconnect with your nutritional wisdom, you might find yourself gravitating toward healthier foods that have the nutrients your body needs. We often hear this about pregnant women eating more beef or other foods they might usually avoid for the nutrient content. This can also happen on a subtler level, and it truly amazes me! How cool is it that your body can communicate with you in that way?

Clearer Skin

The appearance of our skin is often a reflection of what's happening on the inside of our bodies. Considered the largest organ in the body, skin is a living, breathing, and constantly evolving tissue that needs to be nourished to continue doing its important work. Our skin acts as a barrier and is our first line of defense from the outside world. In many ways, it is very similar to the gut: They both are comprised of endothelial tissue; are semipermeable, which allows certain substances to penetrate and keeps others out; and each has its own microbiome. Referred to as the skin flora or the microbiome of the skin, these bacteria communicate with their counterparts in the gut. This communication, or the gut-skin axis, serves as a direct link between the two and is modulated by the immune system.

Dietary choices, nutrient deficiencies, food reactions, hormonal fluctuations, and gut dysbiosis can manifest through the skin: Dry, itchy skin can be a sign of an essential fatty acid deficiency; hormonal acne is commonly seen with excess stress in teenagers and women during their menstrual cycle; food allergies are often reported with redness of the skin or hives; and poor gut health is associated with a slew of skin conditions from acne and psoriasis to eczema and rosacea.

The ways we tend to treat skin issues don't offer long-term solutions. Medication and abrasive skincare products are harmful to the microbiome of both our skin and our gut. They can create a whack-a-mole situation—solving one problem but creating another. Remember, your skin is semipermeable, and chemicals from skincare, makeup, and other beauty products can get into your bloodstream and cause hormonal issues or toxic accumulation. The best path toward a long-term solution is to change the conditions in your body, get to the root cause of the skin ailment, and treat it from the inside out.

Better nutrition, water intake, sleep, gut health, and stress reduction can do absolute wonders for your skin. On The Reset, many people report reduced puffiness, a more even skin tone, fewer blemishes, clearer and brighter eyes, and that elusive "glow." And, if you're looking for nontoxic skincare product recommendations, check out the Resources where I've listed all my go-to brands and products.

Reduce Inflammation

Inflammation is a natural and healthy immune response to infection, injury, or stress. If you've ever had a swollen ankle or a bug bite that got red and puffy, that's inflammation: your immune system's way of treating an infected area or anything else it deems harmful.

While inflammation is an important defense mechanism, too much of it can become problematic; certain foods, pathogens, stress, toxic exposure, injuries, and lack of sleep can all lead to inflammation. Prolonged, or chronic, inflammation develops slowly, and there is a lot of research to support its role in developing chronic diseases like cancer, heart disease, Alzheimer's, type 2 diabetes, and arthritis. When you get a splinter, for example, the inflammatory response is quick and efficient, but chronic inflammation is quiet, often going undetected for years.

Some of the top inflammatory foods include alcohol, sugar, industrial seed oils, factory-farmed meat, and dairy products. These ingredients are in everything from commercial salad dressings and mayonnaise to gluten-free crackers, oat milk, and kombucha, and can be hard to avoid. To combat inflammation, I like to take a two-pronged approach. First, you have to reduce your consumption of inflammatory foods, prioritize sleep, decrease your toxic exposure, and practice stress management techniques. In addition to avoiding these inflammatory behaviors, you need to introduce more anti-inflammatory foods, including spices like turmeric, ginger, cinnamon, and cardamom; healthy fats from olive oil, avocados, fatty fish, nuts, and seeds; fiber from fruit, vegetables, and whole grains; and leafy greens in both variety and abundance. This is precisely what we'll be doing on The Reset while setting you up with the right foods and information to continue these practices when your Reset is complete.

One of the primary sources of inflammation, especially in the United States, is an imbalance between omega-6 and omega-3 fatty acids. These essential fatty acids (EFAs) are considered essential because our body cannot make them, so we must obtain them from our diet. They are important for many biological functions, including cellular structure and messaging, mood and cognition, hormone production, immune function, bone health, and more, but inflammation occurs when they are out of balance.

Omega-6 fatty acids are abundant in seed oils, like canola, safflower, sunflower seed, and soybean oils. They are used in virtually all processed foods and many restaurants because of their affordable price and high smoke point. Omega-3-rich fatty acids come from fatty fish, grass-fed meat, eggs, flaxseeds, chia seeds, avocados, and walnuts. Marine sources have the highest concentration of EPA and DHA, two types of omega-3s that are particularly anti-inflammatory.

On The Reset, we work to achieve an optimal balance of EFAs by simultaneously lowering omega-6 intake and increasing omega-3 intake. We do this by removing processed, fried, and other omega-6-rich foods and adding in more omega-3 sources. We don't need to eliminate all omega-6 food sources—they play a role in our health as well; we just want to ensure we're consuming balanced measures of these EFAs.

Improved Mood & Productivity

When you're well-rested, have sustained energy, and have less stress, inflammation, brain fog, cravings, and digestive issues, you feel *really* good. This will undoubtedly improve your mood, ability to focus and get things done, confidence in yourself, and outlook on life. Practically, you might also feel more inclined to grocery shop, cook, meal prep, or seek out other foods and routines that are supportive of your overall health and well-being. This is when you truly feel the connection between your mind, body, and spirit.

You may finally get the motivation to organize your closet, clean out your pantry, or write those thank-you notes you've been meaning to; maybe you get a request at work that would have ordinarily frustrated and annoyed you, only to find that you're happy to take on the task; or perhaps you move to the front row in your fitness class or finally try that workout you've always been intimidated by. These are the types of actions that feel good long after the moment has passed, and they're contagious; your good energy will rub off on the people around you.

Dr. Bruce Lipton is an expert on epigenetics, which studies how gene expression is influenced by our behaviors and environment, and has done extensive research on how our perception can change our biology. According to Dr. Lipton, our brains are like a paint-by-numbers in reverse; when we see a pretty picture, we paint in happy hormones like dopamine, oxytocin, vasopressin, and growth hormone.[10] These hormones don't just make us feel good but also make us more vibrant and resilient people who are more likely to make healthier choices. On the other hand, when we see a negative picture, our stress and inflammatory responses start firing, leaving our bodies vulnerable.

When we go back to the definition of health as a measure of resilience against disease or injury, the person painting the pretty picture will be more likely to have better health outcomes. So, while improved mood, productivity, and confidence might feel less tangible than some of the other benefits of The Reset we've discussed, in my opinion, it's arguably the most transformative and the one I'm most looking forward to you experiencing.

CHAPTER 4

How to Do The Reset

The Reset is an elimination diet.

We will be removing specific foods for three weeks, then reintroducing them carefully and intentionally so you can better understand your tolerance level and desired relationship with that food. It consists of a simple meal plan, including a protein-rich smoothie for breakfast, a satisfying and balanced lunch, an afternoon snack, and a nourishing dinner.

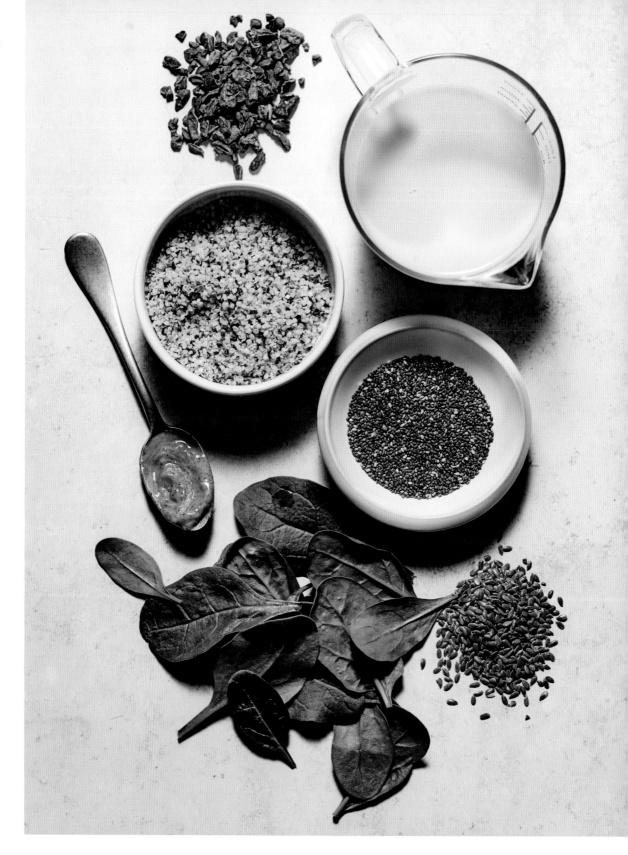

How to Eat

Breakfast: Balanced & Satisfying

Start with a protein-rich smoothie for breakfast. This will fuel your body with the nutrients it needs to stay satiated and energized until lunch. Many of my clients think they will be hungry with just a smoothie for breakfast and are pleasantly surprised by how satisfied they feel after getting adequate protein, fiber, and fat in their morning blends without the influence of excessive blood sugar–spiking sugars. While fruit is an excellent source of nutrition, it also contains sugars. Natural sugars, but sugar nonetheless. A serving of fruit is 1/2 cup. I like to lower that even further in a smoothie to 1/4 cup to curb blood sugar spikes. It's far too easy to turn a smoothie or a snack into a blood sugar bomb, even if we're not using any added sugar besides fruit. Berries like blueberries and raspberries are lower in sugar than fruits like banana, pineapple, mango, and melon.

The recipe section has a whole chapter on Reset-friendly smoothies, or you can create your own concoctions based on the formula in the sidebar.

If it's winter, you live in a cold climate, or are sensitive to colder foods, your smoothie doesn't have to be frozen. Use room-temperature ingredients, or heat your liquids for a warm protein shake. In Chinese and Ayurvedic wellness traditions, cold foods and beverages are thought to slow digestion because they need to be heated to body temperature before digesting. If you like frozen fruit in your smoothie, go for it; if you run cold or struggle with digestion, try something room temperature or warmer.

Reset Smoothie Formula

Protein:
about 15 to 20 grams from protein powder, nuts, and seeds

+

Fat
1 tablespoon nut or seed butter, coconut oil, or 1/4 avocado

+

Fiber
chia seeds, flaxseeds, avocado, cacao nibs, fruits, or vegetables

+

Vegetables
a handful of spinach, kale, zucchini, cauliflower, cucumber, etc.

+

Extras (optional)
fruit, fresh mint, bee pollen, raw cacao, adaptogens, etc.

Juicing fruit robs us of the fiber that helps balance our blood sugar levels instead of giving us a pure shot of fructose. If you like juice, try an all-vegetable juice, and don't treat it as a meal.

Lunch: The Main Attraction

Having lunch as the biggest meal of the day makes digestion at night easier and prevents overeating in the afternoons. Many recipes in this book are perfect for a hearty and filling Reset lunch, but I also love the meal-prep guide (see page 82) for quick and easy assembly of weekday meals.

Vegetables should be the main attraction when constructing your plate, making up at least 50 percent of the dish. This leaves ample room for protein—three to four ounces or about the size of the palm of your hand—and a grain if you choose.

If you need to eat out while on The Reset, try to craft a meal of similar proportions, making sure to avoid gluten, dairy, sugar, fried foods, and processed oils. Salad dressings and sauces are often full of sugar and processed oils; ask for olive oil and vinegar or lemon instead if you aren't sure of the ingredients.

Afternoon Snack: A Mini Meal

The Reset isn't about caloric restriction, and you shouldn't feel starving or go excessively long periods (more than four or five hours) without eating. If you're hungry, eat! Have something substantial, put it on a plate, and enjoy it like you would any other meal. Make sure you get some protein and fats in your snack to keep you full, satisfied, and energized until dinner.

Simple snacks ideas

Hard-boiled egg

Rice cake with peanut butter

Apple with almond butter

Crudité with hummus and seed crackers (see page 193)

Plain, dairy-free yogurt with fruit and nuts

Dinner: Light and Nourishing

On the Reset, the day ends with a warm and nourishing bowl of soup. This easy-to-digest meal is an efficient way to get extra nutrients in while prepping your body for a restful night's sleep. Soup also helps create boundaries to get out of nightly snacking habits and takes some of the guesswork out of what's for dinner.

Ideally, your soup will be pureed for easy digestion, but feel free to keep some texture in your bowl or add garnishes for a little extra crunch. If soup isn't your thing or if you get tired of it, you can switch things up with a smoothie or a meal similar to lunch. If you need to go out for dinner one night or soup doesn't work for you, have protein with vegetables.

Overeating at night is a significant contributor to obesity and other health issues and is generally not an isolated issue but one that comes from the stress, exhaustion, and pressures of daily life. We all know the feeling of plopping down on the couch after a long day at work. It's far too easy to eat a bag of chips or mindlessly overindulge in chocolate. Soup helps bookend your eating window for the day and helps you break out of snacking habits that might be keeping you from your goals.

Eating too close to bedtime can disrupt your sleep by increasing your cortisol levels. Every time we eat, we get a slight increase in cortisol. Sugar, alcohol, and refined carbohydrates will increase this even more and make it difficult to fall or stay asleep. Try to leave at least three hours between dinnertime and bedtime to give your body time to digest its food and allow your cortisol levels to stabilize.

What to Eat

On The Reset, we start with a baseline elimination of gluten, dairy, processed foods, alcohol, and coffee. If you still have digestive or other symptoms after the first week of The Reset, consider other foods or compounds within foods (like naturally occurring chemicals in plants) you may be having a reaction to. And, if you already know that you feel better avoiding a certain food, stay the course. Nutrition at times can include a little detective work. If your symptoms persist, I encourage you to contact a certified nutritionist or healthcare practitioner to help guide your investigation.

FOOD	ENJOY	AVOID
MEAT, POULTRY & FISH	Organic all-grass-fed beef and lamb Pasture-raised pork, poultry, and eggs Wild and responsibly farmed fish and shellfish like salmon, tilapia, pollock, cod, hake, sardines, anchovies, canned tuna, shrimp, oysters, scallops, mussels, clams, and crab	Processed and commercially prepared meat, poultry, and seafood, including sausages, bacon, and deli meats High-mercury fish like shark, swordfish, tuna, marlin, king mackerel, and tilefish
FRUITS & VEGETABLES	All fresh, frozen, or dried fruits and vegetables, organic when possible	Dried fruits with added sugars
PLANT-BASED PROTEINS	All beans and legumes, including organic, non-GMO, fermented soy products (tempeh, miso paste), spirulina, nuts, and seeds	Non-organic, unfermented, and GMO soy products
GRAINS	Whole, gluten-free grains, like brown rice, quinoa, buckwheat, fonio, and millet	Refined grains, like white rice, and gluten-containing grains, like wheat, barley, and rye
DAIRY ALTERNATIVES	Hemp, coconut, and nut and/or seed milk, dairy-free cheeses, and dairy-free yogurts without added sugars	All dairy products, and dairy alternatives with added sugar or processed seed oils
OILS, VINEGARS & CONDIMENTS	All vinegars without added sugar, extra-virgin olive oil, flax, sesame, avocado, and coconut oil, mustard, coconut aminos, gluten-free tamari, mayonnaise made with olive or avocado oil, and unsweetened fruit jam	Processed seed oils, including canola, sunflower, soybean, safflower, peanut, and grapeseed oil, ketchup, relish, chutney, BBQ sauce, teriyaki sauce, conventional mayonnaise, and soy sauce
HERBS, SPICES & SEASONINGS	All herbs and spices	Anything with added sugar or preservatives
SUGAR & SWEETENERS	Stevia, xylitol, and monk fruit extract in moderation	White/brown sugar, high-fructose corn syrup, maple syrup, honey, cane juice, artificial sweeteners, and agave
BEVERAGES	Filtered water, white or herbal tea, sparkling water, green or black tea (one cup per day, max)	Alcohol, coffee, soda, energy drinks, kombucha, and fruit juice

How to Choose Your Foods

There is so much information and confusion about what to eat, and as you dive deeper into the specific categories of food it gets even more confusing. This section provides a deep dive into food sourcing, along with some modification options for your program, if it feels appropriate.

Meat, Poultry & Seafood

From a nutrition perspective, high-quality animal products are an important part of a whole foods diet, which is why they are encouraged on The Reset. Animal protein is the most bio-available source of nutrition, meaning that we can extract and absorb more nutrients from animal products than from plant-based foods. Iron, zinc, amino acids, and certain B vitamins, in particular, are more easily absorbed from animal sources than the same nutrients found in fruits, vegetables, grains, legumes, and other plant foods. That said, how these animals are raised and fed greatly affects the nutrient quality of their meat and their impact on the environment, which ultimately affects our health as well.

If it's not good for the environment, it's not good for our bodies; we are a part of this ecosystem, too, but the debate isn't as simple as eating meat or going plant-based. As they saying goes: *It's not the cow, it's the how.* And while there are undoubtedly a lot of climate and nutrition issues with factory-farmed beef, agriculture practices contribute their fair share to climate change and nutrient depletion as well. Regenerative Organic Certified (ROC) is a certification that holds farms to the highest standards for the health of the soil, animals, and farmworkers. With regenerative farming, plants and animals are farmed together to create more nutrient-rich soil, along with healthier animals and plants for human consumption and more productive soil that is less likely to be affected by extreme weather or contribute to carbon emissions.

Beef

When it comes to beef, look for grass-fed and finished products (labeled *all-grass-fed*), especially from regenerative farms, which not only produces more nutrient-dense meat but also can sequester carbon from the atmosphere and create healthier soil. Most of the damning research and headlines we hear about the environmental and health concerns around beef don't differentiate between meat from cows fed grains like corn and those foraging on grass like they would in their natural habitat. Grass-fed beef is higher in antioxidants, B vitamins, and omega-3 fatty acids, and is naturally leaner and lower in calories;[11] in other words, more nutrient-dense. Grass-fed beef is more flavorful as well. Some report a gamey taste, but that is just the natural taste of beef, and while it can take some getting used to, we should be more concerned about the lackluster taste of factory-farmed beef. Because of grass-fed beef's enhanced flavor and nutrient content, you are likely to feel more satisfied even as you are consuming less.

Factory-farmed cows are often fed a diet of processed grains that have been sprayed with pesticides, which makes them fat and sick. As a precaution, they are given antibiotics to ward off common illnesses and hormones to help further increase their size. This kills their microbiome and changes the nutrient content of their meat and milk. What do you think happens when we eat these products? For one, the meat is much higher in omega-6 fatty acids because of the omega-6-rich feed the cow eats, making it inflammatory. What is potentially even more concerning is that we absorb the antibiotics the cows are given, which can kill our microbiome and make us build resistance if we ever need them. We also consume the hormones that were meant to make the cows fat. I'll leave that one there for you to draw your own conclusions.

A wide variety of meat substitutes have hit the market lately, but they are not perfect solutions. If you want a burger, the best thing you can do for your body and the environment is to find a regenerative, all-grass-fed one. And if beef isn't your thing, just don't eat it. We'll get to plant-based sources of protein, which are absolutely acceptable if you're not a meat-eater.

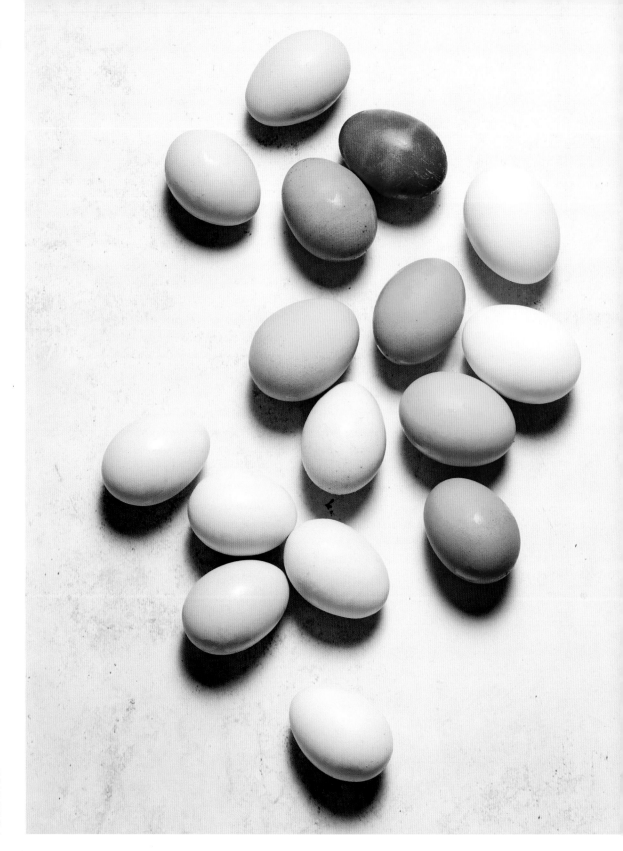

Eggs

Buying and consuming poultry and eggs is similarly nuanced and unnecessarily confusing. How many different terms can they fit on one carton of eggs? One phrase I always look out for is *pasture-raised*. Pasture-raised means the chickens are free to roam and graze on seeds, insects, and worms found on the field, as they would in their natural habitat. Their eggs tend to be higher in iron, omega-3 fatty acids, protein, and antioxidants like vitamins A, E, and C, and lower in saturated fats.[12] One study found that eggs from pasture-raised hens have twice the amount of vitamin E and omega-3 fatty acids, a much higher concentration of vitamin A, and a healthier ratio of omega-6 to omega-3 fatty acids than eggs from commercial hens.[13] Pasture-raised eggs also boast three to six times more vitamin D and are much less likely to carry bacteria like *E. coli*. In fact, you're much more likely to catch a foodborne illness from leafy greens than from an egg.

> Ever notice how some eggs have a pale yellow yolk, and others a bright, vibrant orange one? That's because retinol, a precursor to vitamin A, is bright orange (like a carrot), so the more colorful the yolk, the more nutritious the egg is. When buying pasture-raised eggs, you will get those richly hued yolks we're looking for.

Seafood

We need to be careful about where our seafood comes from for both health and environmental reasons. Sustainable seafood can be wild-caught or responsibly farmed. Ask your local fishmonger or look for third-party certifications like Alaska Responsible Fisheries Management (RMF) and Marine Stewardship Council (MSC) for wild seafood, and Aquaculture Stewardship Council (ASC) and Best Aquaculture Practices (BAP) for responsibly farmed fish. Additionally, it's best to limit your exposure to heavy metals from seafood. Mercury is not the fish's fault; it is released in the air from industrial pollution, accumulates in water, and is absorbed by the fish. Generally, smaller fish have lower levels of mercury, and when larger fish feed on smaller fish, they generate higher mercury levels. Heavy metals impact people differently depending on their age, genetics, microbiome, and toxic load. During The Reset, I want you to avoid bigger fish, like big-eye tuna, swordfish, and tilefish, that are higher in heavy metals as a part of your detox, but in general, most people can consume higher-mercury fish occasionally without adverse health effects. Pregnant or nursing women and young children should avoid high-mercury fish as much as possible.

> When buying fish, think of the acronym S.M.A.S.H., which stands for salmon, mackerel, anchovy, sardines, and herring. These are the healthiest and safest fish to eat; they have low mercury levels, and high amounts of omega-3 fatty acids.

Fruits & Vegetables

All fruits and vegetables are encouraged on The Reset, and, in addition to quantity, I want you to focus on abundance and diversity. The more variety we have in our diets, the more nutrition we get from our foods. When you can, eating regenerative, organic, local, and seasonal will give you better-quality and better-tasting produce. Look into CSA (community-supported agriculture) in your area; it's a great way to support local farms. I understand that this might not be possible depending on where you live, so I've included ideas for sourcing high-quality, seasonal produce in the Resources section.

Buying organic when possible is important to lessen our pesticide exposure. Glyphosate is a pesticide that is widely used in conventional farming practices. Many GMO crops are genetically modified to be resistant to glyphosate, which allows this pesticide to be sprayed right over the crops instead of just the periphery to kill all weeds and other plants interfering with their growth. While we can genetically modify the crops to resist glyphosate, *we* are not resistant to it. Not only is it a carcinogen, but it's also an endocrine disruptor that can affect fertility, the microbiome, liver health, and more.

To be organically certified means that GMO seeds, along with most synthetic fertilizers and pesticides, are not used, and while organic is better, it sadly does not mean pesticide-free. The organic certification is also expensive; many farmers can't afford it, and that extra cost is carried over to the consumer. At my local farmers' market, some vendors are not certified organic but do not spray pesticides. I take them on their word and support them.

If you're concerned about the cost of organic or regenerative foods, check out the Environmental Working Group's website (ewg.org) for their annual Clean Fifteen, Dirty Dozen report, which lists the fifteen fruits and vegetables least contaminated with pesticides and the twelve most contaminated. Avocados, for example, usually rank high on the Clean Fifteen lists because of their thick skin. In contrast, thin-skinned produce, like strawberries and lettuces, are typically found on the Dirty Dozen list. I also love services like Misfits Market, Imperfect Foods, and Hungry Harvest, which deliver irregularly shaped fruits and vegetables that are perfectly nutritious and edible but less desirable for the grocery aisle. It's a great way to save money and help reduce food waste.

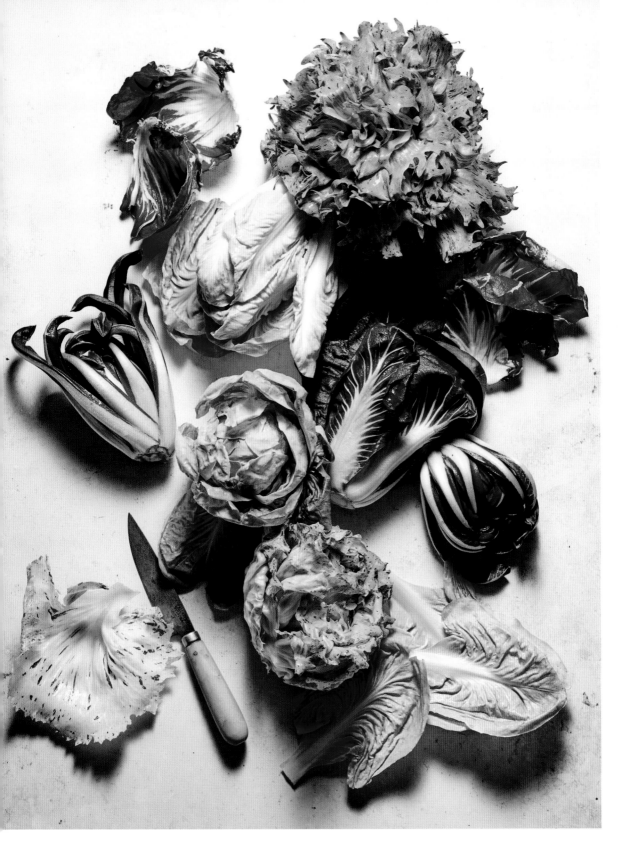

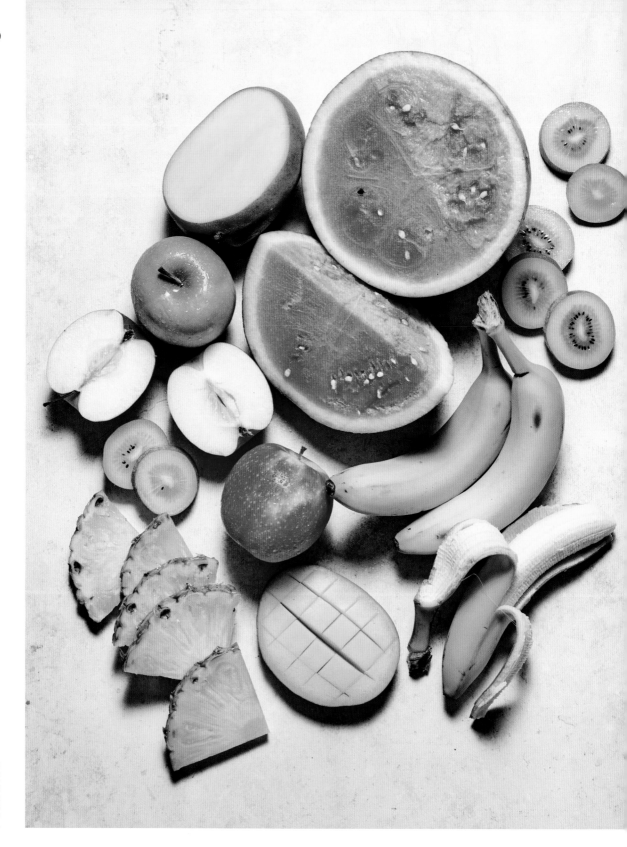

Frozen fruits and vegetables can be a great choice because they are generally picked ripe and frozen straightaway. It can be a more economical and convenient way to increase your fruit and vegetable intake, especially when eating nonseasonal produce. When we buy produce at the grocery store, it sometimes has been in transit for weeks or even months. This means that they are picked before they are ripe, and the longer the fruit or vegetable can ripen on the plant, the more nutrients and flavor it will have. Furthermore, fruits and vegetables start to lose nutrients the longer they live off the vine. If you want blueberries in January, frozen may actually be your most nutritious bet.

As with any type of food, some fruits and vegetables might be off-limits for some people. Cruciferous vegetables, like cauliflower, broccoli, Brussels sprouts, kohlrabi, cabbage, and kale, for example, are incredibly healthy for the vast majority of us. They are excellent for supporting the body's detox mechanisms, lowering inflammation, and even preventing cancer; however, some people will experience painful bloating after eating these vegetables and choose to avoid them. Others will experience symptoms after eating nightshade vegetables or plants with naturally occurring chemicals and compounds like salicylates, lectins, and oxalates. These foods are on the "Enjoy" list of The Reset because they provide valuable nutrition for most, but keeping a detailed food diary will help you connect the dots between any foods you eat and associated reactions so you can dig deeper if your symptoms persist.

Despite their nutrient value, legumes are hard for many people to digest, and you may choose to avoid them on The Reset. That said, if you're vegetarian, legumes are an important source of protein. To make legumes easier on the stomach, sprout and pressure-cook them. I know this can be time-consuming, but luckily, Eden Foods (see Resources) pressure-cooks all their legumes before canning them. I also love the Socca Flatbread recipe on page 138.

Plant-Based Proteins

Most plant-based proteins are not *complete proteins*, meaning that they lack one or more of the nine essential amino acids that our body cannot make. If you don't eat animal protein, try to get *complementary proteins* on your plate, like legumes paired with either a grain, nut, or seed. Many plant-based protein powders are also complete proteins.

Soy is one of the only plant-based foods that is a complete protein. I like whole, fermented soy products, because they are low-carb, easily digested, and contain all the essential amino acids. Soy is also a great source of B vitamins, potassium, magnesium, and fiber, and is a low-glycemic food that helps with blood sugar regulation. That said, soy is one of the most genetically modified and pesticide-laden monocrops on the planet, so limit your intake to organic, non-GMO fermented soy products like miso paste, tamari, and tempeh to reduce toxin exposure.

Peanuts are not a nut but a legume. They are a great source of protein and healthy fats, but it's easy to get fooled into buying peanut products full of added sugars and processed oils. Always check labels on peanut butter (and other nut butters, for that matter) to make sure there aren't any other ingredients besides perhaps a pinch of salt.

Grains

On The Reset, we focus on gluten-free, whole grains. The husk of grains, which is removed when refined, is where all the nutrition is. Protein, fiber, B vitamins, antioxidants, and minerals like magnesium, zinc, iron, phosphorus, and copper are abundant in whole grains, making them a productive food in my book.

Since we're avoiding gluten-containing grains on The Reset, use this as an opportunity to experiment with new and exotic grains. I love black rice (Lemongrass Black Rice, page 135) for its nutty flavor and antioxidant content, and fonio (Mushrooms & Fonio, page 141) for its B vitamins, iron, and resemblance to couscous (which is just tiny pasta!). There are so many wonderful grains and gluten-free alternatives to pasta and bread. Check the Resources section (see page 232) for a list of my favorites.

When consuming grains, we should still be mindful of the blood sugar spike we can get from eating excessive amounts of grain-based foods, refined or whole. To reduce your carbohydrate load, keep your serving size to ½ cup, and when making rice or pasta dishes, invert the ratio of grain to everything else. A pasta dish usually is at least 75 percent pasta with some sauce or toppings, but if you make the dish 75 percent vegetables, sauce, and protein with 25 percent grain, you still get to enjoy that warm bowl of pasta, with more nutrition and less of a blood sugar spike!

Dairy Alternatives

While dairy products might not be a total no-no for you in the long run, discovering your tolerance level to them is an important part of The Reset. When swapping for dairy alternatives, be mindful of the ingredients, especially added sugars and inflammatory oils. Ideally, plant-based milks will have very few ingredients. I've listed my favorite brands in the Resources section, but they may vary by region, so it's important to know what to look out for.

Oat milk, although it foams like dairy milk products, is not the healthiest milk substitute, in my opinion, and should be avoided on The Reset. Oat milk is essentially a juiced grain, which causes a blood sugar and insulin spike. Many oat milks also contain rapeseed oil, which is another word for canola oil. And to add insult to injury, oats are a monocrop, like corn and soy, so even if it's organic, these monocrops are not great for the environment. I prefer an organic, unsweetened nut, seed, or coconut milk with limited ingredients. Generally (and there are some exceptions to this) the non-dairy milks you find in the refrigerated section will be less processed than shelf-stable alternatives. You can always make your own as well. Check out some fun non-dairy milk recipes on page 222.

If ordering something at a coffee shop, like a matcha or another non-coffee drink, ask about their milk options. The barista blends typically need something like sugar or oil for the milk to foam, so if you want an unsweetened version, you have to ask for it.

Oils, Vinegars & Condiments

Cooking oils, vinegars, and condiments are excellent ways to add flavor and nutrition to meals, but can include inflammatory ingredients, like sugar, industrial seed oils, and other additives. Use The Reset as an opportunity to replace these items in your pantry with healthier alternatives; luckily, there are many of them.

Avoiding inflammatory seed oils when cooking is easier than you might think. Extra-virgin olive oil is my oil of choice. I love its flavor and nutrient content, and when olive oil is fresh and high quality, it can be used for cooking up to 400°F. When buying olive oil, look for organic extra-virgin, unrefined olive oil. Bottling and expiration dates are always an important sign, and storing olive oil in an opaque jar helps protect the integrity of the olive oil, which naturally denatures with time and UV exposure.

For a more neutral cooking oil, use avocado oil, which has an even higher smoke point of 520°F. You can also use unrefined coconut oil for cooking if you prefer, but personally, I like avocado oil because it is tasteless, and coconut oil sometimes leaves a coconutty taste to the dish.

It becomes more difficult to avoid processed seed oils when eating out or buying packaged foods. Chips, crackers, and other snack foods are often cooked or fried in canola or other seed oils because they are cheap and have high smoke points. If you want something crunchy on your Reset, I've listed some brands that use avocado, olive, or coconut oil in the Resources section, but remember, these are often not nutrient-dense foods, even if they're healthier than a more processed alternative. When we eat nutrient-poor foods, we feel unsatisfied. This is why it's shockingly easy to eat an entire bag of chips and still feel hungry.

Condiments and commercial salad dressings are generally heavily processed, and high in sugar and inflammatory oils. One of the main ingredients in ketchup, for example, is high-fructose corn syrup, and mayonnaise is a canola oil bomb. You can buy your favorite condiments from brands that use better-quality ingredients like Primal Kitchen, Sir Kensington, and Chosen Foods when eating at home (see Resources).

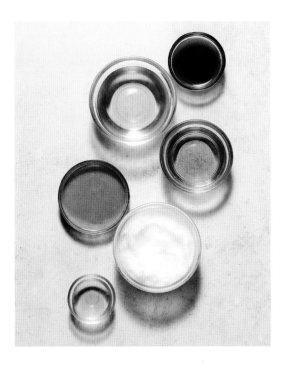
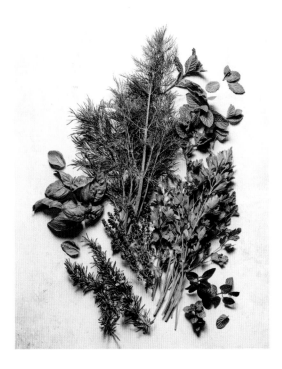

Herbs, Spices & Seasonings

You'll notice that many, if not most, of the recipes in this book use some sort of herb, spice, or seasoning, and I hope this will be an opportunity for you to discover new flavors and ways to jazz up ordinary meals quickly. Herbs and spices are a fantastic way to add nutrition and flavor to an otherwise simple meal, and I recommend using them with abundance on and off The Reset.

There has been a lot of negative talk about salt, or sodium, in recent years, but it is an essential mineral that is vital for your health and makes food more palatable. In fact, I am often more concerned about a lack of sodium with my clients than too much. Too little sodium can lead to increased cravings for sugar and refined carbohydrates, decreased energy, weight gain, insulin resistance, high blood pressure, and more.

Sodium is an important electrolyte, alongside other minerals like calcium, magnesium, and potassium, which regulates the fluid balance in the body, and plays a crucial role in nerve and muscle function. Processed foods are often extremely high in sodium and lack these other minerals, but when eating a whole foods diet, you will get more of these essential minerals to help maintain optimal fluid balance in the body.

Sugar & Sweeteners

For many, one of the most profound benefits of The Reset is getting a handle on sugar consumption. Sugar is addictive and doesn't offer much nutrition. It can be a hard cycle to break out of, which is why we're being diligent in reducing sugar consumption on The Reset.

Sugar can easily hide in even the least suspicious of foods, like frozen organic sweet potato fries, savory sauces, gluten-free bread, and more. Some additional terms for "sugar" include syrup, malt, nectar, and anything ending in -ose (like dextrose, fructose, and maltose). The American Heart Association's recommendation for daily sugar consumption is less than 24 grams for women and 36 grams for men;[14] for reference, the average scoop of ice cream has 27 grams of added sugar, and that doesn't include the cone or the toppings. Make sure to diligently check labels for added sugars when grocery shopping and doing your pantry cleanout.

Aside from a few natural sugar alternatives and fruit, sugar in any form (including honey and maple syrup) is not included in The Reset. Stevia, xylitol, and monk fruit extract are acceptable sweeteners, and while they don't cause a blood sugar spike, they should still be used sparingly.

On The Reset, we are aiming for 0 grams added sugar, but whether you're doing The Reset or not, I like to set a limit to less than 10 grams of total sugar for any packaged foods.

Beverages

Drinks are an easy way to consume excess stimulants, like coffee and sugar, and often provide little to no nutritional value. Sometimes, however, drinking plain water just doesn't cut it, so I've provided some recipes to make your water more exciting and palatable (see page 228) and included some drink suggestions in the Resources section.

Hidden sugars pop up in seemingly healthy drinks, too. We talked about non-dairy milks, but kombuchas can also contribute to unnecessary sugar intake and should be avoided on The Reset, along with juices made with fruit. Try sparkling water or iced tea instead. Beware of diet drinks as well, which contain chemical artificial sweeteners. These sweeteners can be inflammatory and dangerous, and still train us to want more sweet-tasting foods, even if they don't have calories or cause a blood sugar spike.

If you drink alcohol, The Reset is the perfect opportunity to reevaluate your relationship with it. Many of my clients have never gone twenty-one days without drinking in their adulthood, and while moderate alcohol consumption can be a part of a healthy lifestyle, taking a break will allow you to understand how it affects you and why you reach for it. Has a nightly glass of wine become a crutch for you, or do you overdo it on the weekends and feel sluggish the next day as a result? While alcohol is often used to help us wind down, it can disrupt your sleep, blood sugar, and hormones, leading to nutrient deficiencies and increased anxiety.

Cutting coffee while on The Reset is the part of the program I get the most resistance to. And don't get me wrong: Coffee is not bad for you. It is actually a great source of antioxidants, but it is easy to become overly dependent on it or turn it into a dessert (cue the vanilla latte). Furthermore, it can make some people nervous, anxious, and restless, and contribute to digestive issues. You may be surprised to discover your natural energy is just as potent as caffeine without any side effects. I have a coffee-free month once a year, and I begrudge it for a few days each time. So, if you're wincing, I'm with you, but trust me, it's not as bad as you think. The first few days off coffee can be rough—headaches and fatigue are normal, but that's all the more reason not to be so dependent on it, and I can assure you that you will find your natural energy quickly. It's not forever, just three weeks! Feel free to enjoy a cup of green tea, which has a much milder amount of caffeine and is loaded with nutrients.

CHAPTER 5

Getting Started

Before you begin your Reset, make sure to take at least a few days to prep, buy ingredients, and familiarize yourself with the recipes and principles of the program.

If these concepts feel unfamiliar or overwhelming to you, or if this is your first time doing The Reset, you may want to take a week or more to get into the swing of things. Here are a few ways to mentally and physically prepare yourself in the leadup to your Reset.

One trap I often see people getting into is perfectionist thinking. As they say, don't let perfect be the enemy of the good. Perfectionist thinking is an all-or-nothing, on-the-wagon off-the-wagon mindset that holds many people back from reaching their goals and finding sustainable routines they can stick with. When our expectations are higher than we can realistically maintain, we set ourselves up to fail. Be realistic about your goals. Instead of saying, "I'll never eat sugar again," you could reframe your goal to: "I'm going to work on decreasing my sugar intake, reading labels more diligently, and managing my blood sugar levels more to decrease cravings and sugar intake." This is a way more achievable goal, with actionable solutions to keep you motivated!

Goal Setting & Motivation Check

I'm a big believer in goal setting and manifestation, but in order to achieve our goals we need tangible motivators to get us there. Start thinking about what motivated you to pick up this book or to try The Reset and write it down. Then, think of three to five things you could actively do to get yourself there. For example, I've had the forever goal of being able to do a handstand. In order to get there, I need to make a commitment to practicing yoga three or more times a week, working on my shoulder mobility by doing daily exercises, and improving my core strength by doing plank exercises. In the pursuit of my handstand goal, I stay motivated by more immediate and tangible benefits like the high I get after a class, the socialization aspect of seeing my yoga friends, feeling stronger in my core, and experiencing less back and neck pain. Another goal might be to improve the health and appearance of your skin. Your daily motivators could be the energy you get from drinking more water, improved digestion from a daily probiotic habit, or developing an interest in clean beauty to replace your conventional skincare products (which I recommend doing one-by-one as they run out to lessen the economic blow).

Check Your Calendar

Take a look at your calendar and try to find a time when you can really focus and commit to doing The Reset properly. I don't want this program to be unnecessarily stressful because of work, familial, or social obligations. There are workarounds for the occasional dinner out, but try to start at a time when you can chill. If you have a wedding to attend, travel plans, or a big work event, that might not be the best time for it.

Make a Plan

Set yourself up for success by planning out your first few days of meals. Go grocery shopping, do some meal prep, and maybe even write down exactly what you plan to have for breakfast, lunch, snack, and dinner each day. You won't need to be this thorough for the duration of The Reset, but it helps to get you started.

You may also want to experiment with smoothies or try other recipes so you have some solid options you know you like before you start. This will make things easier, especially if you're not used to preparing your own meals or if some of the ingredients are unfamiliar.

Start Weening Off Coffee, Sugar & Alcohol

Slowly ween off coffee, sugar, and alcohol in the week leading up to your start date. Consider cutting down to one coffee a day if you normally drink more, ordering half-caff instead of full caffeine, or switching to a caffeinated tea drink like matcha or Earl Grey. This will help ease any caffeine withdrawals you might have in the first few days of your Reset. As tempting as it might seem, don't go overboard on alcohol or sugar in the days leading up to your Reset. You will likely feel tired for the first few days, and a sugar- or alcohol-induced hangover just makes it worse.

Snap Some Photos

On your first day, or just before, take some pictures of your face and body. Change can be subtle, especially when you're living with yourself day in and day out. It's nice to have a record to compare day one to day twenty-one.

Schedule Reset-Friendly Activities

Think of some fun activities you can do on The Reset to replace dining out. Maybe it's a picnic lunch, a hike, or a movie with friends. Pick up some good books; schedule self-care practices like massages, manicures, or facials; book workout classes; plan a museum visit; or try something new like reiki, acupuncture, or, my favorite, cupping. If you can recruit a friend or partner to do The Reset with you, it will make these activities even more enjoyable!

The Reset is also great for when you have a big work or school project on your plate. You will feel your stamina, productivity, and energy levels skyrocket, so it's a great help to dig into any work you might need to do.

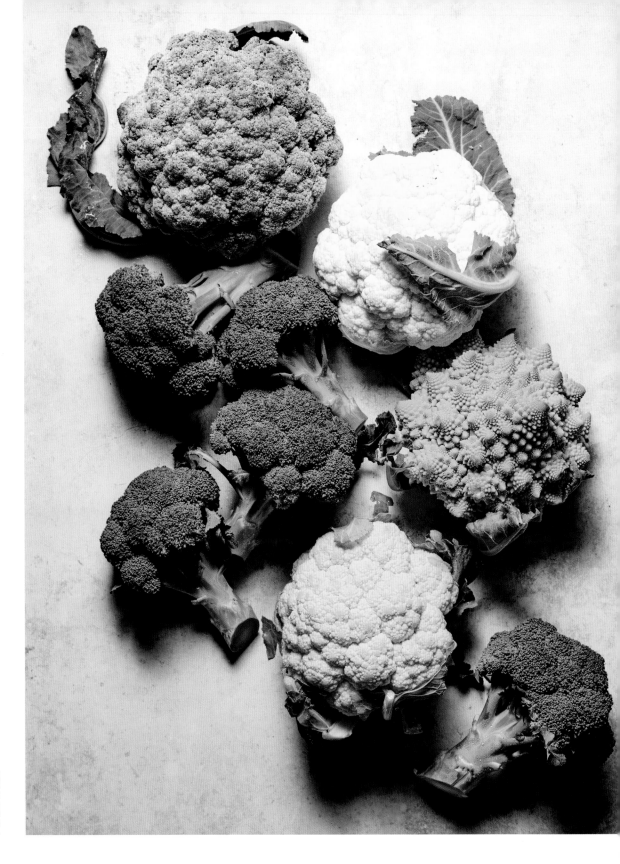

Optimize Your Reset

Incorporate these healthy-living tips and tools into your Reset, and perhaps some will carry over into your post-Reset routine.

1. Eat More Vegetables

When it comes to vegetables, more is more! Aim to increase not just the amount of vegetables you eat, but also variety. Each vegetable has its own mix of vitamins, minerals, and phytonutrients, so the more diversity in your diet, the more nutrition you get. Try for seven servings (a serving is equal to a cup) of vegetables a day, and aim to make your meals at least 50 percent vegetable-based. Be mindful of starchy vegetables like potatoes, squash, and peas, because they have a higher carbohydrate load and glycemic index. You don't have to avoid them altogether; they are still a great source of nutrition, but make sure you're consuming more non-starchy vegetables like leafy greens, broccoli, and zucchini.

For a little extra credit, try the **twenty-vegetable challenge** by eating twenty different vegetables through the course of your Reset. This might seem like a lot at first, but individual lettuces (spinach, romaine, arugula, kale, etc.), herbs (basil, cilantro, dill, mint, etc.), garlic, onion, and ginger all count! You might be surprised how this exercise encourages you to try new foods and get creative. It's one of the many ways that a nutrient-rich diet can be more flavorful and exciting.

2. Try Intermittent Fasting

If you sleep, you fast. That's actually where the word *breakfast* comes from; you're literally *breaking* your *fast*. Intermittent fasting can sound daunting, but it starts with just a twelve-hour window between dinner and breakfast. It is a simple and effective tool for weight management, blood sugar stabilization, hormone regulation, immune support, and cellular repair. Many of us intermittent fast intuitively, but being more consistent with it and, potentially, stretching that window will give you more significant benefits.

Digestion requires a lot of energy and coordination in the body. When you're fasting, your body can allocate those resources to other functions, like cellular repair. This is important for reducing oxidative stress, eliminating toxins, keeping your immune system healthy, and improving biomarkers for disease.

Fasting can help increase insulin sensitivity, which regulates hunger and fat storage, and also increases the amount of human growth hormone (HGH), an important hormone that builds muscle, burns fat, increases bone density, improves

In addition to intermittent fasting, pay attention to the timing of your meals. Ideally, meals are spaced three to five hours apart. This allows your **migrating motor complex (MMC)** to activate. The MMC is like a broom sweeping undigested food through your gastrointestinal tract, and is important for proper digestion. If you're hungry less than three hours after a meal, by all means eat, but ask yourself why so you can make adjustments moving forward. Did you not have enough protein, fiber, or fat in your last meal, or did you have too much sugar or a meal high in carbohydrates? And perhaps you aren't hungry, but thirsty, bored, stressed, or procrastinating on something instead. When you go longer than five hours without eating, you run the risk of getting overly hungry and overeating. So, if lunch is at noon and dinner is at seven, make sure you schedule a substantial snack in between!

your sleep, elevates your mood, and even reduces signs of aging. It is also a great tool to help you become more aware of your hunger cues, manage cravings, and bookend the day to prevent mindless snacking. Additionally, studies show that fasting can improve cognitive function, especially when it comes to learning and memory.

Our metabolism thrives on a cycle of daytime eating and nighttime rest. Eating late at night can increase the risk for obesity and diabetes and disrupt our circadian rhythm.[15] To optimize your Reset, try an earlier dinner (or eat only during daylight) to allow more time for digestion before bed. While this is ideal, I recognize that it's not always possible, and simply sticking with a fasting window will still provide many benefits.

So, how long should you fast? I am thrilled with a twelve-hour fast; personally, that's all I do most days. That means, if you finish dinner by 7:30 p.m., wait until at least 7:30 a.m. to have breakfast. I love intermittent fasting because you can decide on a schedule that works for you; and it doesn't have to be static. If you have a late dinner one night, just have a later breakfast the next day. If you want to take it further, you can increase your fast to fourteen, sixteen, or even eighteen hours. I find this especially effective for men and postmenopausal women, but again, twelve hours is fantastic.

While you're fasting, you can still have water, tea, or other drinks without calories. The most important thing is to listen to your body. If fasting makes you hungry and miserable, don't do it. And if you're not sure, ask your doctor. Pregnant and nursing women, along with anyone with fertility issues or who has experienced disordered eating, should not intentionally fast—many people will still naturally do the twelve hours, which is fine.

3. Drink Water

The daily recommended water intake is half your body weight in ounces, but drinking enough water is a struggle for many. Hydration is important for your mood, sleep, energy levels, regulating body temperature, immune function, detoxification, skin health, getting nutrients to cells, lubricating joints, and more. If you have a hard time drinking water, use your Reset as an opportunity to focus on making a habit of it that will hopefully carry on to your post-Reset routines. From natural flavorings, electrolyte powders, and carbonation to water bottles, home filters, and phone reminders, simple tools can significantly increase water intake. Try to avoid drinking water in plastic (even plastic water filters) as that can increase your toxin exposure. Check out the Hydration Station recipes (see page 228) for tasty water alternatives, and the Resources section for other ways to jazz up your water intake.

4. Practice Mindful Eating

How often are you doing other things while you're eating? When we're distracted, we lose the connection to our food, which can impair digestion, impact the absorption of nutrients, or lead to overeating. Digestion begins in the mouth, so remind yourself to chew and not rush your meals. Try to sit down for all your meals and snacks, preferably without the interference of your phone or the TV, and take the time to truly enjoy your food.

5. Prioritize Your Sleep

Develop a nightly routine that is consistent, calming, and sets the stage for a good night's rest. This can start with turning off all screens at least thirty minutes before bed and following a ritual that winds you down for the day. Maybe that means a bath, a special skincare regime, cozy pajamas, reading a book, or doing a meditation. Try to set a vibe with music, a noise machine, or essential oils.

What you do during your waking hours can make a huge impact on your sleep as well. The Reset's meal plan of nutritionally balanced meals with protein, fiber, and healthy fats at regular times helps regulate your hormones and circadian rhythm to improve the quality of sleep.

6. Eat One Fermented Food a Day

Fermented foods like miso paste, sauerkraut, kefir, and kimchi are excellent sources of probiotics and great for gut health. Part of the gut healing protocol of The Reset is to reduce foods that aggravate gut health, and increase consumption of gut-friendly foods. The Miso Caesar Salad (see page 107) is a staple for me, and I love snacking on an unsweetened non-dairy yogurt with fruit and nuts while on The Reset. You can also find lots of different fermented vegetables at the grocery store. I particularly love fermented carrots as an addition to salads, or just by the forkful.

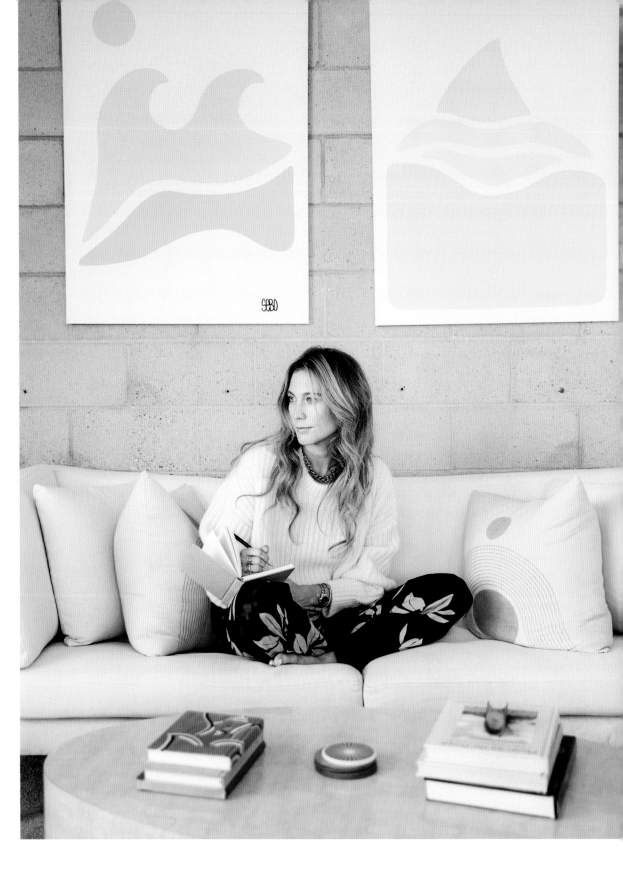

7. Keep a Journal

The practice of journaling during The Reset not only provides a record of change and data surrounding your habits, but it is also a great exercise in mindfulness and accountability. The idea of journaling isn't to scrutinize or feel shame around your food choices but to develop a deeper understanding of how certain foods and behaviors affect you, positively and negatively. As you'll see in the prompt below, make sure to log more than just what you ate. How you slept, if you exercised, your mood, digestion, and any other observations will help document your journey and provide valuable insights. Be detailed; it will be interesting to see how your habits and routines have changed through the course of The Reset. It may feel subtle at the time, but it's these little shifts that make the biggest difference, and a lot can change in three weeks.

Journal Prompt

How are you feeling today?

How did you sleep last night?

How much water did you drink today?

Did you exercise?

Breakfast (time/food/drink):

How did you feel after breakfast?

Lunch (time/food/drink):

How did you feel after lunch?

Dinner (time/food/drink):

How did you feel after dinner?

Snacks (times/foods/drinks):

How did you feel after snacking?

8. Develop a Supplement Routine

A multivitamin is like an insurance policy. While I always like to look toward food first, we have no realistic way of knowing how much nutrition is in what we eat, and sadly our poor soil health doesn't guarantee nutrient-density. This is where a multivitamin comes in; it's not a substitute for a healthy diet but rather an assurance that you're getting all the vitamins and minerals you need to function optimally.

There are a few supplements I think most people should be taking: a multivitamin, omega-3 fatty acids, probiotics, and magnesium.

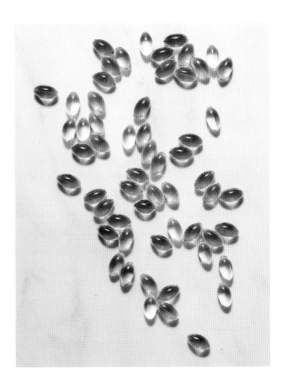

To get the recommended amount of omega-3 fatty acids, you would have to consume about twelve ounces of fatty fish per week (that's about three to four servings). Most people don't eat this much seafood, so it makes sense that many people are deficient in this essential nutrient. Marine sources of omega-3 fatty acids are full of EPA and DHA, two highly anti-inflammatory compounds. When we consume omega-3s from non-marine sources like walnuts, flaxseeds, and avocados, we only convert a small amount of those omega-3s into EPA and DHA.

The research into omega-3 fatty acids and their health benefits is staggering. Benefits of omega-3s include improved mental health and sleep; fewer and less painful menstrual cramps; improved cognitive function (particularly for pregnant women and infants), skin health and appearance, and cardiovascular and eye health; and reduced risk of obesity, age-related illnesses like Alzheimer's and dementia, metabolic syndrome, cancer, ADHD, and asthma in children.

When it comes to mental health, studies show that omega-3 supplementation can help treat and prevent depression; this includes postpartum depression in new mothers and lowering the risk of depression in the mother's offspring. Additional studies have found that omega-3s can help lower anxiety, and there is even a correlation between this essential fatty acid and the reduction of crime in prisons.[16]

Many adults are lacking in this essential nutrient, but luckily omega-3 supplements and foods are generally safe and well-tolerated, making it an excellent treatment and prevention method for inflammation, cognitive health, and mood disorders. My recommendation for most people is to eat fatty fish regularly and take an omega-3 supplement. Vegans who don't want to consume any fish-derived products can get a marine algae omega-3 that is 100 percent vegan and full of the EPA and DHA that we're looking for!

A probiotic helps create and maintain a healthy microbiome, or balance of bacteria in the gut. I used to be on the fence about the benefits of a probiotic as an everyday supplement, but over the years, I've seen the depletion of our soil health and prevalence of toxins from the environment, food, water, medication, and other sources mount enough evidence for me to recommend most people take a probiotic. In addition to taking a probiotic, look to add prebiotic-rich foods to your diet; these are foods for the good bacteria in your gut and include plant-based foods like asparagus, garlic, onion, bananas, leeks, and chicories.

Magnesium is involved in more than three hundred biochemical reactions in the body, including immune health, bone health, nerve and muscle function, energy production, digestion, and stress management. Studies suggest that up to 50 percent of the US population is magnesium deficient, but my guess is that it's a lot higher than that. I run nutrient tests for most of my clients, and I have never seen a result (mine included!) that didn't show an increased need for magnesium.

If you are on medication, pregnant, nursing, or have a genetic disorder, your needs might differ. It's always a good idea to check with your doctor or a certified nutritionist before taking any supplements.

Vitamin D3 is the most bioavailable form of vitamin D, and it's important for our immune system, mental health, bone density, hormone function, and more. Sunlight is our primary source of vitamin D, but even if you live in a sunny climate, you probably spend lots of time in doors, covered up, and lathered in sunscreen. Combining D3 with K2 helps with bone density.

9. Move

Exercise is essential not just for muscle building, calorie burning, and cardiovascular health, but also for digestion, stress management, and mental health. In fact, I think the mental and cognitive benefits of exercise outweigh the physical ones. This means that you don't need to do a super strenuous workout to get the benefits. Try to do something active every day of your Reset, whether it's a walk, light stretching, or more rigorous exercise like a spin class.

Weight training is an important part of any exercise routine. Building muscle does more than make us "toned." The more muscle we have, the more glycogen stores we have. Glycogen is a form of glucose. When our blood sugar levels are high, insulin directs the body to store excess glucose (or sugar) in the liver, muscle, and fat tissue. When we have more muscle, more of that glucose will be diverted to our muscle stores rather than our fat stores. Think of it like a buffer that helps us maintain a healthy weight.

Building muscle mass also increases our total daily energy expenditure, which is the amount of calories our body burns in a day. After the age of thirty, we start to lose muscle mass, about 3 to 5 percent per decade, making it increasingly important to do weight-bearing activities as we age. To build and maintain muscle, try to work out so you feel sore once a week, and make sure to prioritize protein in your diet.

You can still do The Reset if you prefer more vigorous exercise or are training for something. Increase your protein intake by adding an additional snack or having a higher-protein dinner—either something similar to lunch, added protein in your soup, or a protein smoothie. As always, listen to your body. If you need more, have more.

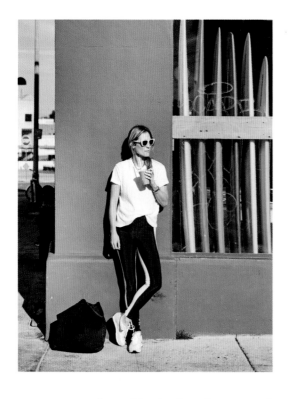

10. Get Outdoors

Spending time outside, especially in nature, is hugely beneficial for your mental and cognitive health. Many of our hormones are influenced by sunlight. Vitamin D (which is actually a hormone, not a vitamin) is an essential nutrient that our body creates from sun exposure and is integral to our physical and mental health. It plays a key role in boosting your mood, and deficiencies of this nutrient are linked to an increased risk of depression. Only 10 percent of our vitamin D is obtained from food; the rest comes from sun exposure and supplementation when sun exposure is unavailable.

Our production of happy hormones, like endorphins and serotonin, increases when we spend time outdoors; this stimulates the activity of our parasympathetic nervous system, which is responsible for feelings of calmness and relaxation, and lowers blood pressure and heart rate. Melatonin is a hormone that plays a crucial role in sleep regulation and our circadian rhythms. Lack of sun exposure can increase melatonin production and make you feel drowsy in the afternoon. Just a few minutes outside, even on a cloudy day, will block melatonin production, so you have more energy during the day and feel sleepy when you should—at night!

Ever get an afternoon productivity slump? This is often when people crave stimulants like sugar and caffeine to get them through the day. But, just going for a walk outside can improve your working memory, which helps with concentration and focus. If you have a long to-do list and no time for a walk, think again. Maybe you don't have time not to.

Ideally, we would be spending two or more hours outside every day. I understand this might not be realistic for everyone (or most!), but maybe you can increase your time outdoors by eating meals outside instead of indoors, taking work calls or exercising outdoors, or walking instead of driving places when possible. Urban dwellers can take advantage of city's parks, sit by a window (hopefully with a view of trees), and get indoor plants to bring the outdoors in.

11. Self-Care

It always amazes me how we tend to reward ourselves with things that aren't good for us like desserts, alcohol, or other indulgent foods (I am guilty of this, too!). What if we substituted those rewards with things that were truly of benefit to our bodies? I lived in Hong Kong for several years in my late twenties and early thirties and love how many Eastern cultures prioritize self-care. Massages are seen as hugely beneficial for your health, maintaining strong relationships, and excelling at work; acupuncture treatments, reflexology, and other traditional Chinese medicine modalities are considered a vital part of one's healthcare regimen and are much more accessible than they are here in the United States. A dear friend's mother once told me that I need to get regular massages or I will be mean to my husband. Of course, this made me laugh, but I think about this often, because she is not wrong! Use your Reset as an excuse to take care of yourself, and create some rituals you can continue after your program is complete.

And as much as I love a trip to the spa, it's important to note that self-care isn't always a glamorous and doesn't always have to involve an expensive facial. True self-care can be hard work; it's going to the doctor for regular checkups, balancing your checkbook, flossing your teeth, going to bed early, and making time to grocery shop and prioritize healthy meals.

Most of the recipes in this book fit into The Reset, and some are just a delicious way to expand your repertoire. I encourage my clients to mix and match the recipes that sound best to them, and you should, too! But if you would like a little more guidance, sample menus and meal plans follow to help you begin the process of figuring out how The Reset best fits into your life.

Meal-Prep Guide

Cook once, assemble later. Here is a quick guide for making easy weekday meals at home by prepping a few things ahead of time. With a couple of pre-prepared bases, vegetables, proteins, and sauces, you can have multiple salad and bowl options. If you're doing The Reset, add one to two soups to your weekly meal prep and freeze the leftovers so you can have more variety.

Bases

Make sure you have one to four base options to make salads, pastas, and bowls.

Leafy greens: I recommend always having two varieties in the refrigerator, like spinach and arugula. Prewashed, store-bought greens work great.

Grains: Make some brown rice or quinoa, or try one of the below recipes.

Mushrooms & Fonio (page 141)

Herbed Brown Rice & Cauliflower Pilaf (page 139)

Sweet potato: Baked whole, in slices, or as fries (page 000)

Pasta: Cook the whole box and store in the refrigerator to make quick pasta dishes. See resources section for gluten-free brands.

Bread: Find some gluten-free alternatives you like, or try these recipes.

Socca Flatbread (page 138)

Nut & Seed Protein Bread (page 191)

Vegetables

Prepare at least two vegetable options. They can be simple sliced, steamed, or sautéed vegetables, or one of the below recipes.

Meal-Prep Roasted Vegetables (page 129)

Spiced Carrot Salad (page 120)

Spicy Roasted Broccoli Rabe (page 114)

Proteins

Prep one and have two to three other easy proteins ready to go for the week.

Poultry: You can roast a whole chicken, cook parts of a chicken, buy a rotisserie chicken for the week, or try one of these recipes.

Chicken en Papillote (page 156)

Spiced Chicken with Green Olives (page 161)

Zaatar-Crusted Chicken Cutlets (page 155)

Meat: Simply grilled meats make great leftovers.

Mediterranean Lamb Meatball Lettuce Wraps (page 162)

Shepherd's Pie with Celery Root Top (page 158)

Eggs: Breakfast dishes make quick, easy, and healthy lunches and dinners as well.

Hard-Boiled Eggs with Dipping Salts (page 193)

Seafood: If getting fresh seafood is a logistical challenge for you, try frozen so you can incorporate more into your weekly meals.

Roasted Salmon with Cherry Tomatoes & Shallots (page 175)

Shrimp & Veggie Pad Thai (page 148)

Legumes: Make sure to have canned or dried beans at the ready as an easy plant-based protein option.

Dressings & Sauces

Always have a couple flavorful sauce and dressing options. I recommend making one each week in addition to having some premade sauces and dressings at home.

Miso Caesar dressing (page 107)

Carrot-Ginger Dressing (page 130)

Pistachio Pistou (page 220)

Premade dressings (see Resources)

Extras

Want to add some extra flair to your meals? Make or stock up on these pantry flavors to bring your meal-prepped dishes up a notch.

Pickled Red Onions (page 210)

Garlic Chili Oil (page 216)

Brazil Nut Romesco (page 218)

Preserved Lemons (page 217)

Tomato Confit (page 211)

Olives

Meal-Prep Dish Examples

Mix and match your meal prep to make original bowls and salads.

Spicy Salmon Salad: Harissa Salmon + mixed greens + Spicy Roasted Broccoli Rabe + Pickled Red Onions + Socca Flatbread

Chicken Pesto Bowl: Chicken en Papillote + Meal-Prep Roasted Vegetables + sautéed spinach + Herbed Brown Rice and Cauliflower Pilaf + pesto

Mediterranean Lamb Meatball Salad: Lamb Meatballs + Quinoa and Arugula Salad + Crispy Smoked Paprika Chickpeas + Tahini Dressing

Lunch Eggs: Scrambled eggs + Tomato Confit + arugula salad + lemon + shallot olive oil + a slice of Nut & Seed Protein Bread

Ready-to-Go Dishes

You may also want to make extra of certain dishes you love to have leftovers later in the week. Here are great recipes for batch cooking.

Chicken, Peanut, & Soba Noodle Salad (page 144)

Fusilli with Braised Chicken Thighs, Mushrooms, Spinach, & Sun-Dried Tomato Pesto (page 145)

Shepherd's Pie with Celery Root Top (page 158)

Turkey Lettuce Wraps (page 152)

Snacks

If lunch and dinner are more than five hours apart, you are going to want to fit a snack in between. Here are some snack ideas that will keep you going to dinner.

Apple + nut butter

Hummus + crudités + Seeded Crackers (page 193)

Nut & Seed Protein Bread (page 191) + Chocolate-Hazelnut Spread (page 212)

Unsweetened non-dairy yogurt + berries + high-protein cereal (see Pantry in Resources section)

Hard-Boiled Eggs with Dipping Salts (page 193)

Dark chocolate + berries + cashews

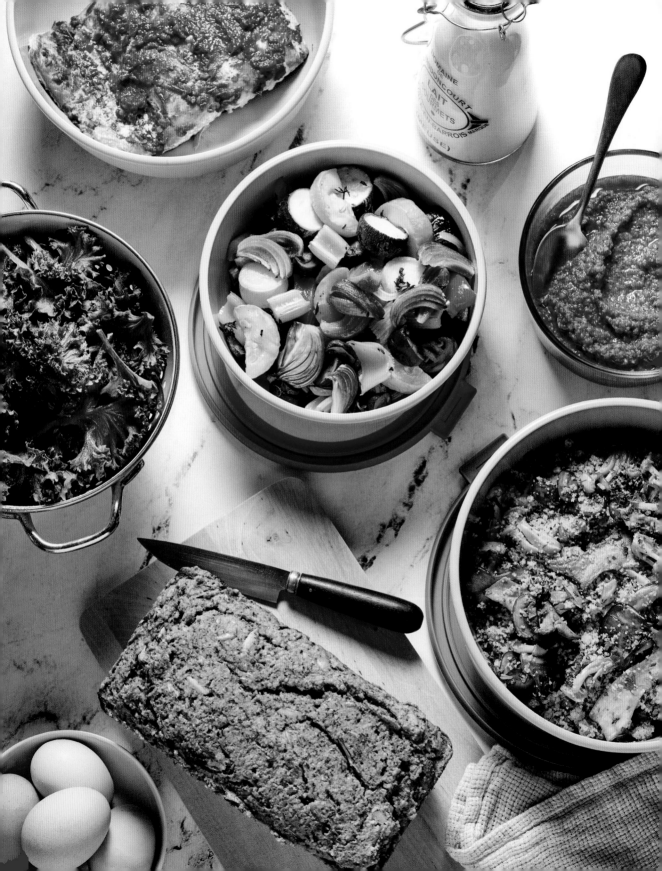

A Day in The Reset
Sample Menus & Meal Plans

Here are some ideas of what you can have on The Reset using recipes from the book. To cut back on cooking and prep time, repeat your favorite dishes or lean on easy meals from the meal-prep plan.

	BREAKFAST	LUNCH	SNACK	DINNER
DAY 1	Mint–Chocolate Chip Smoothie (page 93)	Green Goddess Salad (page 109)	Hard-Boiled Eggs with everything bagel salt (page 193)	White Bean & Leek Soup (page 178)
DAY 2	Cucumber-Vanilla Smoothie (page 95)	Miso Caesar Salad (page 107) + Chicken en Papillote (page 156) + avocado	Apple + almond butter	Harissa Salmon (page 165) + Spicy Roasted Broccoli Rabe (page 114)
DAY 3	Chocolate-Covered Cherry Smoothie (page 99)	Garlicky Kale Frittata (page 100) + Simple Green Salad (page 124)	Nut & Seed Protein Bread (page 191) + Chocolate-Hazelnut Spread (page 212)	Jazzy Carrot & Parsnip Soup (page 181) + Seeded Crackers (page 193)
DAY 4	Supreme Green Smoothie (page 96)	Shrimp & Veggie Pad Thai (page 148)	Carrot-Apple Snack Muffin (page 207)	West African Peanut Soup (page 188)
DAY 5	Golden Smoothie (page 98)	Fusilli with Braised Chicken Thighs, Mushrooms, Spinach & Sun-Dried Tomato Pesto (page 145)	Banana Bread (page 201) + almond butter	Blueberry-Basil Smoothie (page 99)

CHAPTER 6

Reintroduction

By the end of The Reset, you should be feeling *really* good and deeply connected to your nutritional wisdom.

The goal, however, is not to avoid the eliminated foods indefinitely, but rather empower yourself with the knowledge of how these foods truly affect you and wipe the slate clean on any dependencies on sugar, processed foods, alcohol, or caffeine you may have developed prior to The Reset. Now that you've set your new baseline and done some serious self-discovery, use your intuition to build a harmonious and loving relationship with the foods you eat, align your actions with your goals, and eat in a way that is not only immensely satisfying and filling but also helps you achieve and maintain your desired health outcomes.

Try not to rush back into your pre-Reset routines. Spend a week or so slowly reintroducing the foods you've eliminated one by one. This is a golden opportunity to see how a particular food actually makes you feel. Start with what you suspect you might have the highest intolerance to; note any symptoms you might experience, like fatigue, irritability, digestive issues, or a rash. If you don't notice any effects, move down the list, introducing a new food every thirty-six to forty-eight hours. Continue to journal throughout this process, monitoring your digestion, energy levels, mood, and sleep until you've reintroduced all the foods on your list.

When reintroducing gluten and dairy, you may want to take a phased approach, because some will have more or less of a tolerance to certain forms of these foods. For gluten, start with organic sourdough bread or a sprouted wheat bread like Ezekiel, then move on to pasta and more commercially prepared gluten-containing foods. With dairy, begin by reintroducing fermented forms of sheep's or goat's milk like yogurt or cheese. If this feels okay, move on to cow's cheese or yogurt, and lastly, reintroduce milk products.

So, What's Next?

The recipes in the next section of this book are not just for The Reset, but for life! They are low-glycemic, plant-forward, full of adequate protein, fiber, fat, vitamins, minerals, phytonutrients, and more. But most important, they're delicious everyday meals easy enough for Tuesday nights, yet fun enough for a dinner party with your dearest friends. These are recipes that will help you continue on your wellness journey, even if your partner, kids, or anyone else you cook for doesn't share those same goals. Remember, what you do the majority of the time is more impactful on your health than what you eat the minority of the time. So, by eating this way at home, you will be reinforcing the healthy habits you developed during The Reset.

Over time, some of your old habits inevitably will start to creep back in: one coffee a day turns into three; you might start craving sweets, eating more processed foods, or drinking more alcohol; you may notice your mood or energy levels declining, your clothes may start to feel tight, your skin may break out, or you may feel some digestive discomfort. This is your signal to Reset! Whether it's seven, ten, or twenty-one days, come back to these principles to Reset and take your wellness journey a step further.

My husband and I have been doing The Reset together since we first met, which is ten years as of the publication of this book. Without fail, we do it every January and sporadically throughout the year when we feel like we're slipping out of the healthy habits that make us feel good and function at our best. We are entrepreneurs and parents and literally cannot afford to feel sluggish or anxious. We know that this is just the tool we need to put some pep in our step. And it works. Every time.

To me, food freedom isn't just eating what I want, it's being in control of it. While I love coffee, wine, cookies, and ice cream, I don't want to be beholden to them, or feel like I *need* them. This program has absolutely changed my life. It's given me the ability to feel great in my skin and confident in my food choices, and it's freed up my mental energy to stress less about what I'm eating and focus on my family, friends, work, and the things that make me happy. I cannot wait to see how your Reset empowers you.

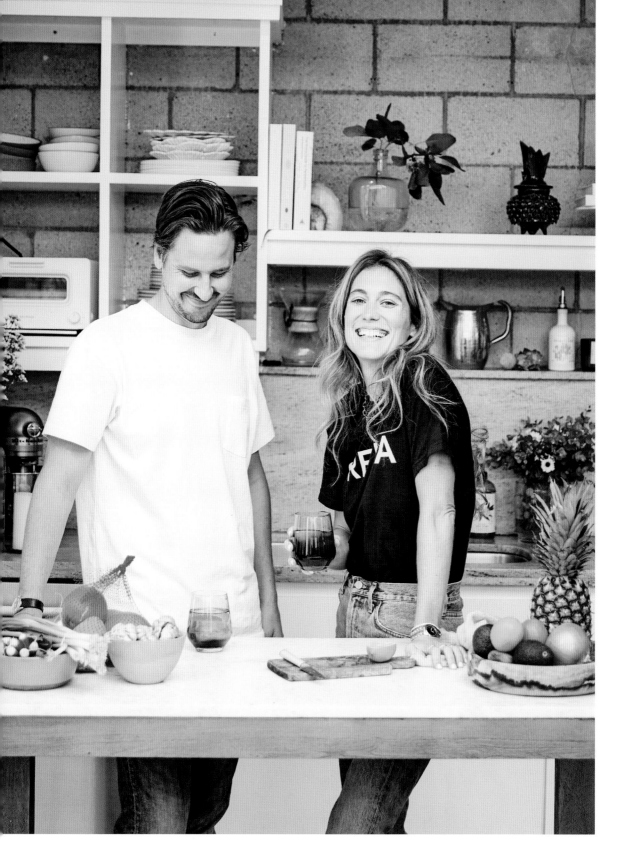

PART 3

RECIPES

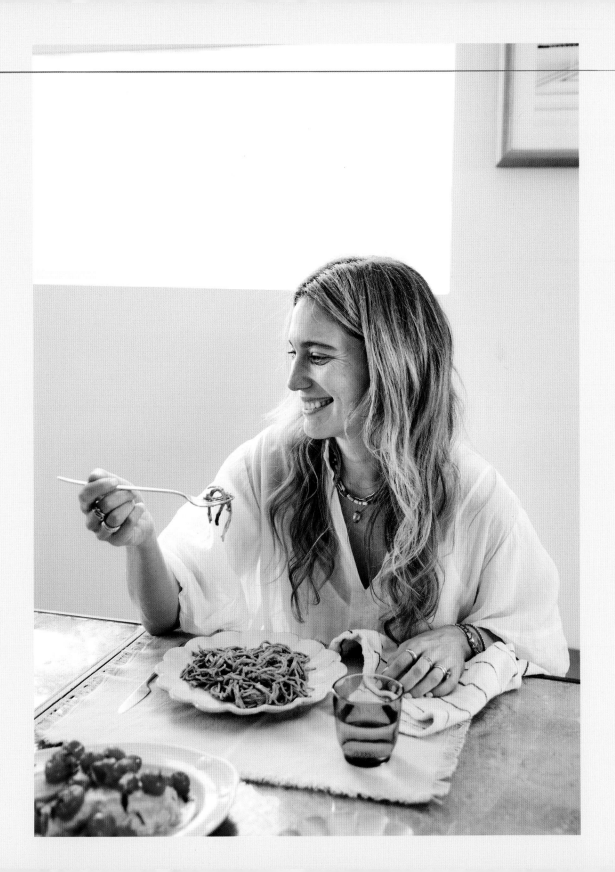

Smoothies
& Breakfast

Mint–Chocolate Chip Smoothie

This is hands down my favorite smoothie recipe, and my go-to whenever I'm not sure what to make for breakfast. I love it because it's flavorful, not overly sweet, and has two sneaky vegetables and an herb! Don't be dismayed by the zucchini; it's surprisingly undetectable and makes this shake extra creamy.

SERVES 1

1 scoop vanilla protein powder

½ cup spinach

¼ medium zucchini

3 to 5 sprigs fresh mint

1 tablespoon almond butter

1 tablespoon chia seeds

½ tablespoon unsweetened cacao nibs

1½ cups dairy-free milk, filtered water, or a combination of the two

In a high-speed blender, add the protein powder, spinach, zucchini, mint, almond butter, chia seeds, cacao nibs, and dairy-free milk. Blend until smooth.

Sesame-Cardamom Smoothie

Cardamom is one of my favorite spices. It is slightly sweet and most definitely pungent, but beyond its flavor profile, cardamom is known for its anti-inflammatory and digestive-supporting properties. I love the pairing of cardamom with the cinnamon, ginger, vanilla, and tahini in this smoothie; it's a satisfying, vibrant, and soothing start to the day.

SERVES 1

1 scoop vanilla protein powder

⅛ teaspoon or a pinch of ground cardamom

¼ teaspoon ground cinnamon

1 tablespoon tahini

¼ cup cauliflower, frozen or fresh (riced cauliflower also works)

¼ banana, fresh or frozen

1 thumb-size piece fresh ginger, peeled, or 1 teaspoon ground ginger

1½ cups dairy-free milk, filtered water, or a combination of the two

¼ teaspoon white sesame seeds (for garnish)

In a high-speed blender, add the protein powder, cardamom, cinnamon, tahini, cauliflower, banana, ginger, and dairy-free milk. Blend until smooth. Garnish with sesame seeds.

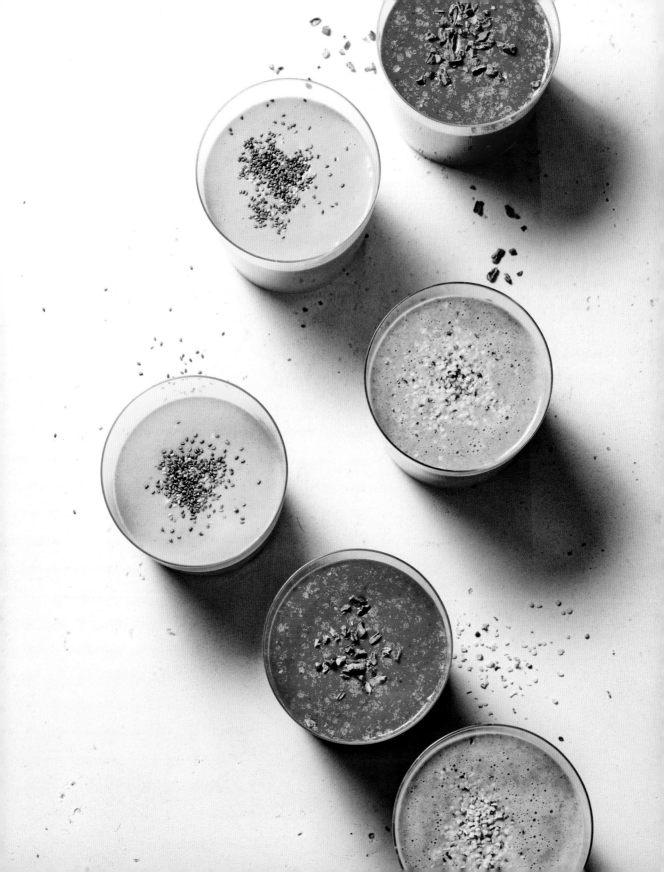

Cucumber-Vanilla Smoothie

I first discovered a cucumber smoothie at a juice shop in Los Angeles, and it quickly became a favorite ingredient of mine. As unusual as it may sound for a smoothie, cucumber lends a fresh and energizing kick to this morning blend. I especially love this during the warm summer months.

SERVES 1

1 scoop vanilla protein powder

1 cup spinach

½ medium English cucumber, sliced (about ½ cup)

1 tablespoon almond butter

1 tablespoon chia seeds

1½ cups dairy-free milk, filtered water, or a combination of the two

In a high-speed blender, add the protein powder, spinach, cucumber, almond butter, chia seeds, and dairy-free milk. Blend until smooth.

Pumpkin Pie Smoothie

Pumpkin-spiced-everything lovers, this one is for you! Pumpkin pie will always be my favorite dessert, and this smoothie gives me all the fall feels without the excess sugar.

SERVES 1

1 scoop vanilla protein powder

¼ cup canned pumpkin puree

1 tablespoon coconut butter

1 thumb-size piece fresh ginger, peeled, or 1 teaspoon ground ginger

1 teaspoon ground cinnamon

1½ cups dairy-free milk, filtered water, or a combination of the two

In a high-speed blender, add the protein powder, pumpkin, coconut butter, ginger, cinnamon, and dairy-free milk. Blend until smooth.

Supreme Green Smoothie

This smoothie captures the refreshing essence of a green juice, but with the added benefits of the fiber and nutrients found in the whole vegetable, rather than just the juice.

SERVES 1

1 scoop vanilla protein powder

¼ avocado, peeled and pit removed

1 teaspoon matcha powder

½ cup spinach

1 thumb-size piece fresh ginger, peeled, or 1 teaspoon ground ginger

½ celery stalk

1 tablespoon lemon juice

1½ cups dairy-free milk, filtered water, or a combination of the two

In a high-speed blender, add the protein powder, avocado, matcha powder, spinach, ginger, celery, lemon juice, and dairy-free milk. Blend until smooth.

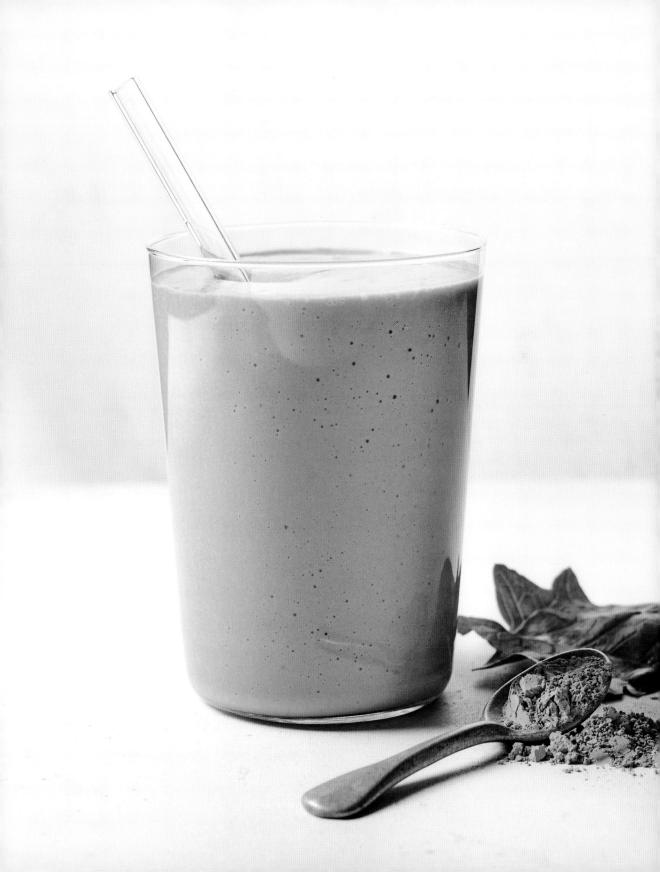

Golden Smoothie

If you live in a cold climate or are sensitive to cold temperatures, this smoothie is great served warm. Just heat up the milk before you blend for a soothing golden shake.

SERVES 1

1 scoop vanilla protein powder

1 teaspoon ground turmeric

1 thumb-size piece fresh ginger, peeled, or 1 teaspoon ground ginger

¼ cup cauliflower, fresh or frozen (riced cauliflower also works)

1 tablespoon almond butter

1 tablespoon flaxseeds, ground or whole

1½ cups dairy-free milk, filtered water, or a combination of the two

In a high-speed blender, add the protein powder, turmeric, ginger, cauliflower, almond butter, flaxseeds, and dairy-free milk. Blend until smooth.

Raspberry-Beet Smoothie

Beets may feel like an unusual breakfast ingredient, but from a nutritional standpoint, they're an excellent food to start the day with, and they pair well with sweet and tangy raspberries. High in nitrates (not the additive, the natural kind), beets can help widen the blood vessels to reduce blood pressure and improve exercise performance and brain function; they're also a hydrating source of fiber, which helps with digestion.

SERVES 1

1 scoop vanilla protein powder

¼ cup raspberries

½ medium-size cooked beet, or 1 small beet, halved

1 tablespoon coconut butter

1 tablespoon unsweetened cacao nibs

1½ cups dairy-free milk, filtered water, or a combination of the two

In a high-speed blender, add the protein powder, raspberries, beet, coconut butter, cacao nibs, and dairy-free milk. Blend until smooth.

Chocolate-Covered Cherry Smoothie

Instead of using vanilla protein powder and raw cacao powder, you could simply use chocolate protein powder, but in my experience, the combination of vanilla protein powder and raw cacao powder gives a better chocolate flavor.

SERVES 1

1 scoop vanilla protein powder

¼ cup frozen cherries

½ tablespoon raw cacao powder

1 handful spinach

1 tablespoon almond butter

1 tablespoon chia seeds

1½ cups dairy-free milk, filtered water, or a combination of the two

In a high-speed blender, add the protein powder, cherries, cacao powder, spinach, almond butter, chia seeds, and dairy-free milk. Blend until smooth.

Blueberry-Basil Smoothie

Coconut butter is an excellent source of both fat and fiber. While coconut oil is an extraction of the oils from the coconut meat, coconut butter is a puree, much like a nut butter; it has a much higher fiber content and a sweet, nutty taste.

SERVES 1

1 scoop vanilla protein powder

¼ cup blueberries, fresh or frozen

1 tablespoon coconut butter

1 handful spinach

3 to 5 fresh basil leaves

1 tablespoon chia seeds

1½ cups dairy-free milk, filtered water, or a combination of the two

In a high-speed blender, add the protein powder, blueberries, coconut butter, spinach, basil, chia seeds, and dairy-free milk. Blend until smooth.

Garlicky Kale Frittata

Frittatas are a versatile recipe every cook should have in their repertoire. They're great for brunch with friends or meal prep for a busy week. Enjoy as a quick breakfast or Reset lunch with a side salad (it pairs great with the Simple Green Salad on page 124) and a slice of toast. Feel free to use this recipe as a template and play around with different vegetables. Some other combinations I love include cherry tomatoes and basil, sautéed mushrooms and leeks, and asparagus.

SERVES 6

3 tablespoons extra-virgin olive oil, divided

4 garlic cloves, minced

1 bunch kale, washed, stems removed, leaves roughly chopped

1 tablespoon lemon juice

Sea salt

8 large eggs

¼ cup full-fat coconut milk

Freshly ground black pepper, to taste

1. Preheat the oven to 350°F.

2. In a 10-inch cast-iron skillet or an oven-safe frying pan, heat 2 tablespoons of the olive oil over medium heat.

3. Add the garlic, and sauté over low heat until soft and fragrant, 3 to 4 minutes. Add the kale, lemon juice, and a pinch of salt, and continue to sauté until the kale is wilted, 5 to 6 minutes.

4. Remove the kale from the skillet and place in a bowl. Set aside.

5. In another bowl or measuring cup, combine the eggs and coconut milk, along with a generous pinch of salt, and whisk until fully incorporated and frothy.

6. In the same skillet, heat the remaining tablespoon of olive oil, then add the egg mixture. Cook over medium heat for 3 to 5 minutes, then spread the kale mixture evenly over the eggs.

7. Cook over medium heat until the edge of the frittata starts to pull away from the pan, about 5 minutes. Transfer the skillet to the oven and cook for 10 to 15 minutes more, or until the eggs are completely set. You should be able to give the skillet a good shake without the eggs jiggling.

8. Season to taste with pepper and serve immediately, or keep in the refrigerator for up to 5 days.

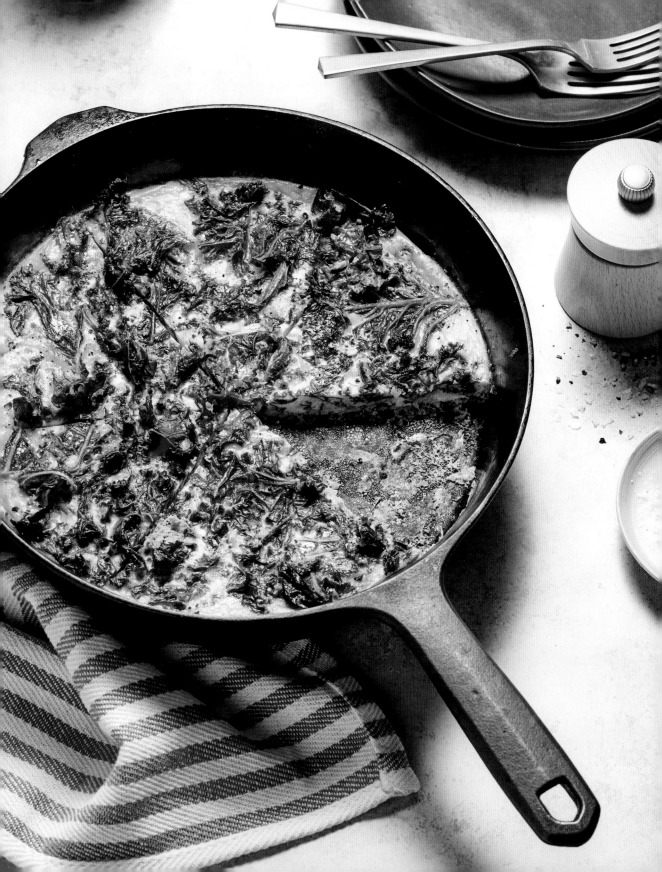

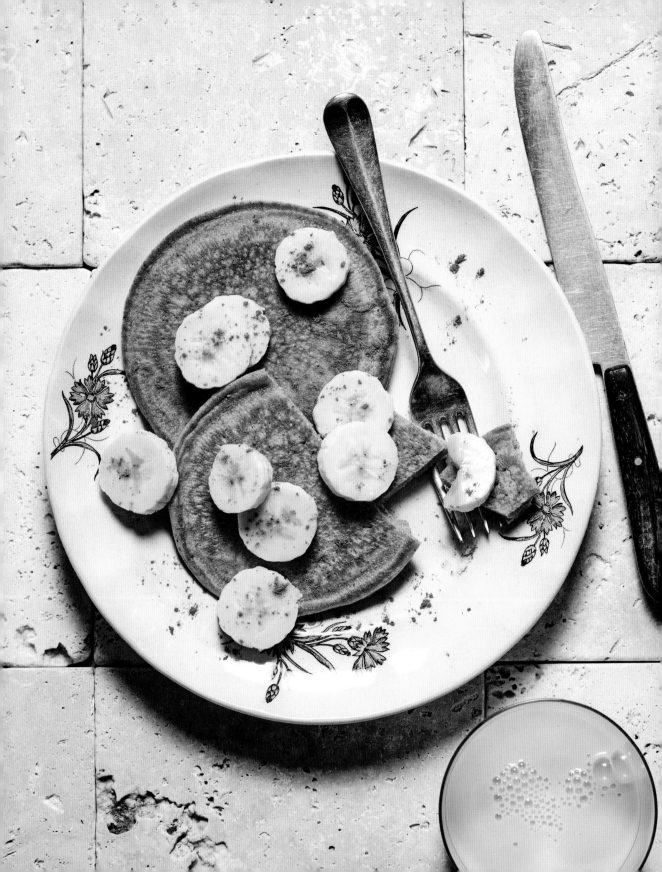

Almond-Banana Pancakes

I started making banana pancakes for my son when he was a baby, and of course I would end up eating half of them each morning. These are a little bit more of a grown-up version, but still totally appropriate for kids!

MAKES 4 PANCAKES

1 very ripe banana, plus 1 banana, sliced (optional)

2 eggs

2 tablespoons almond butter

½ cup gluten-free all-purpose flour

¼ teaspoon ground cardamom

Pinch of sea salt

Blueberries and/or chocolate chips (optional)

1 to 2 tablespoons avocado oil, plus more as needed

1. In a high-speed blender, combine the banana, eggs, almond butter, flour, cardamom, and sea salt. Blend until smooth. Add in the blueberries, chocolate chips, and/or sliced banana, if using, and blend until smooth.

2. In a medium-size frying pan over medium-high heat, heat ½ to 1 tablespoon of the avocado oil. Add one-quarter of the pancake batter to the pan. Allow to cook for 2 to 3 minutes, then flip and cook 2 to 3 minutes more.

3. Transfer the pancake to a plate and repeat with the remaining batter, adding more avocado oil as needed.

Grain-Free Hot Cereal

This low-glycemic oatmeal alternative packs a nutritional punch with a plethora of fiber, protein, healthy fats, and nutrients to keep you full and satisfied until lunch.

SERVES 2

¼ cup coconut flour

2 tablespoons white chia seeds

2 tablespoons ground flaxseeds

2 tablespoons unsweetened coconut flakes

2 scoops vanilla collagen powder

¼ teaspoon ground cinnamon

2 cups dairy-free milk

Fresh berries (for serving)

Nut butter (for serving)

1. In a small saucepan, add the coconut flour, chia seeds, flaxseeds, coconut flakes, collagen, and cinnamon and whisk to combine.

2. Add the dairy-free milk and cook over medium-low heat, whisking continuously until it thickens and the milk has been absorbed.

3. Serve with fresh berries and a drizzle of your favorite nut butter.

Vegetables & Salads

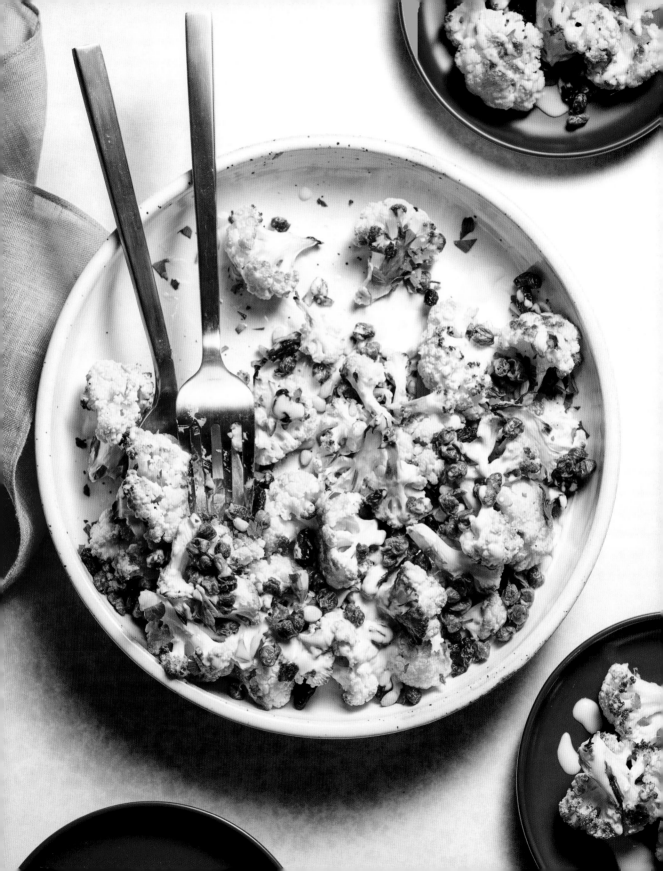

Roasted Cauliflower with Popcorn Capers, Pine Nuts & Tahini Dressing

Popcorn capers will be your new favorite side dish accessory, and I'd highly encourage you to lift this part of the recipe for other vegetable preparations; they are crispy, tangy, salty, and delicious. Since they are just simmered in olive oil, they aren't deep-fried, but they taste like they are (which is why we like them!). Dry your capers as much as you can before adding them to the hot oil to prevent splattering.

SERVES 4

1 head cauliflower, cut into florets

6 tablespoons extra-virgin olive oil, divided

Sea salt and freshly ground black pepper, to taste

¼ cup capers, drained

2 tablespoons tahini

1 tablespoon water

2 tablespoons lemon juice

¼ cup raisins

¼ cup pine nuts, toasted

½ cup chopped fresh parsley

1. Preheat the oven to 375°F and line a baking sheet with parchment paper.

2. In a large bowl, add the cauliflower florets, toss with 2 tablespoons of the olive oil, and season generously with salt and pepper.

3. Arrange the cauliflower on the prepared baking sheet and bake for 35 to 45 minutes, or until cooked through and golden brown. Browning is key to this dish, so if your cauliflower isn't sufficiently brown after 45 minutes, continuing roasting in 2- to 3-minute increments until it is.

4. While the cauliflower is cooking, make the popcorn capers and dressing. In a medium sauté pan, heat 2 tablespoons of the olive oil over medium heat. Pat the capers dry with a paper towel. Add the capers to the pan and allow them to cook until crisp, 3 to 5 minutes. Remove the capers with a slotted spoon and place them on a paper towel–lined plate.

5. To make the dressing, in a small bowl, whisk together the tahini, water, and lemon juice. Slowly whisk in the remaining 2 tablespoons of olive oil. Season with salt and set aside.

6. Remove the cauliflower from the oven and add it to a serving bowl.

7. To the bowl with the cauliflower, mix in the raisins, pine nuts, and parsley. Drizzle the tahini dressing on top and garnish with the popcorn capers.

Miso Caesar Salad

This salad is great for entertaining alongside a simple roast chicken and rice, but the dressing is easy enough to make for an everyday lunch. I often just add the ingredients into a cup, whisk with a fork, and drizzle over greens, leftover protein, and avocado. A simple yet exciting five-minute lunch.

SERVES 2 TO 4

1 tablespoon miso paste

2 tablespoons water

Juice of ½ lemon

1 tablespoon Dijon mustard

¼ cup extra-virgin olive oil

6 to 8 cups torn little gem or romaine lettuce (from 2 to 4 heads)

¼ cup walnuts, toasted

Note: You can store this dressing in the refrigerator for up to 5 days. Loosen with some water (½ tablespoon at a time), as it will thicken slightly as it sets.

1. In a small bowl, add the miso paste, water, and lemon juice, and whisk to combine. Whisk in the Dijon mustard.

2. Slowly whisk in the olive oil, continuing to whisk until fully incorporated.

3. In a large mixing bowl, toss the lettuce with the dressing. Transfer to a large salad bowl or individual bowls and top with the toasted walnuts.

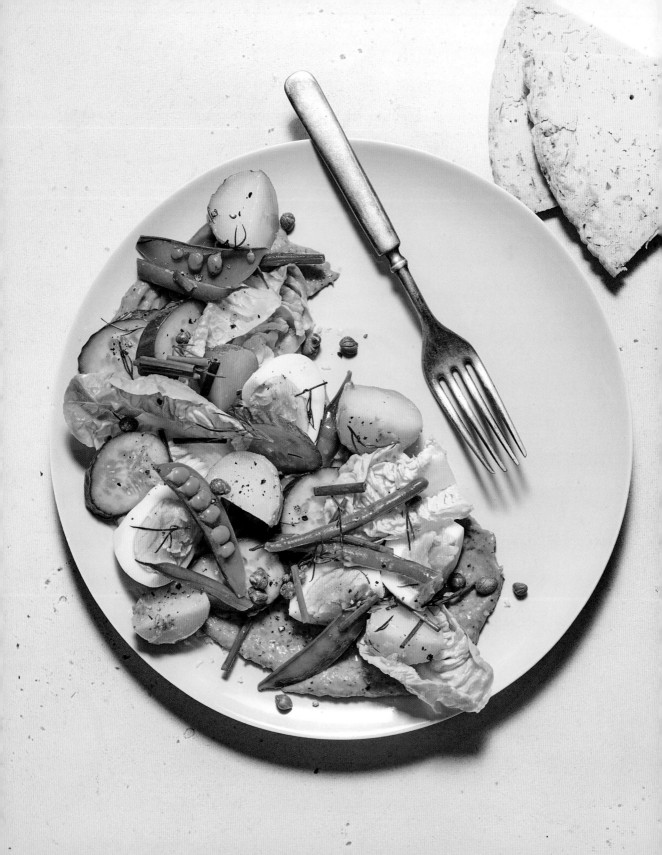

Green Goddess Salad

Full of fresh greens, vibrant herbs, and zesty capers, this salad is like spring in a bowl, and is perfect for lunch alfresco. Save any extra dressing you might have and use it as a dip for crudités and crackers.

SERVES 2

½ **medium zucchini**

¼ **ripe avocado, peeled and pit removed**

2 **tablespoons capers, drained, divided**

¼ **cup fresh basil leaves**

¼ **cup fresh dill, plus more for garnish**

1 **tablespoon fresh tarragon leaves**

½ **tablespoon tahini**

¼ **cup fresh lemon juice**

¼ **cup plus 1 tablespoon extra-virgin olive oil**

2 **tablespoons filtered water**

Sea salt to taste

1 **head little gem lettuce, leaves torn or separated**

1 **Persian cucumber, sliced**

8 **to** 10 **haricot verts, steamed**

8 **to** 10 **snap peas, steamed**

3 **to** 4 **new potatoes, boiled**

4 **hard-boiled eggs**

3 **to** 4 **fresh chives, diced**

1. In a food processor, combine the zucchini, avocado, 1 tablespoon of the capers, basil, dill, tarragon, tahini, lemon juice, ¼ cup of the olive oil, water, and a pinch of salt. Blend until fully combined. The dressing can be made 1 day in advance.

2. When ready to serve, toss the lettuce with the remaining tablespoon of olive oil and a pinch of salt.

3. Divide the dressing between two shallow bowls or plates, spreading evenly across the bottom of the dish.

4. Arrange the lettuce, cucumber, haricot verts, snap peas, new potatoes, and hard-boiled eggs over the dressing.

5. Garnish with the remaining tablespoon of capers, chives, and a sprinkle of salt.

VEGETABLES & SALADS

Winter Citrus Salad with Crispy Shallots

The sweetness of the orange juice in the dressing, paired with shallot olive oil, crispy shallots, and creamy pine nuts, is the perfect pairing. I love this salad so much that it makes me look forward to winter! Don't skimp out on the Crispy Shallots & Shallot Olive Oil recipe on page 215. It brings this dish to life. And don't fret if you can't find kumquats or blood oranges. They have a very specific season and can easily be substituted with extra navel orange segments.

SERVES 4

1 tablespoon whole grain
   mustard

1 tablespoon orange juice
   (see Note)

2½ tablespoons Shallot Olive
   Oil (page 215), divided

Sea salt to taste

1 head radicchio, quartered
   and leaves torn

1 blood orange, segmented

1 navel orange, segmented

4 to 6 kumquats, sliced in
   rounds

1 tablespoon toasted pine nuts

½ cup chopped fresh parsley

1 cup Crispy Shallots (page
   215)

Note: Use the leftover juice from the segmented navel orange.

1. In a small bowl, whisk together the mustard and orange juice, then slowly add 2 tablespoons of the shallot olive oil and a pinch of the sea salt. Set aside.

2. In a large bowl, mix the radicchio and the remaining shallot olive oil together with a pinch of salt.

3. On a serving platter or in a serving bowl, layer the radicchio, blood orange, navel orange, kumquats, pine nuts, and parsley.

4. Drizzle the dressing over the salad and top with the crispy shallots.

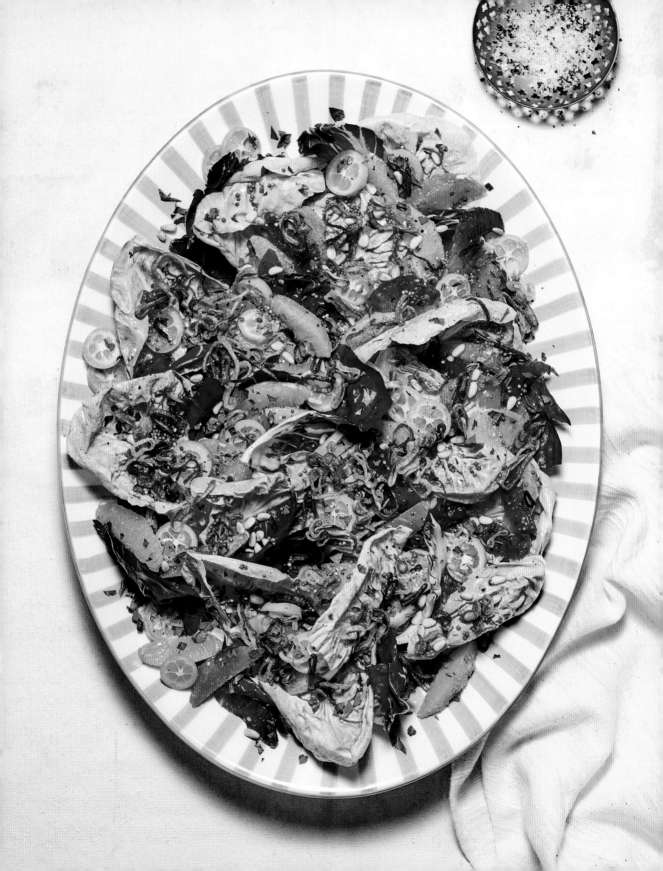

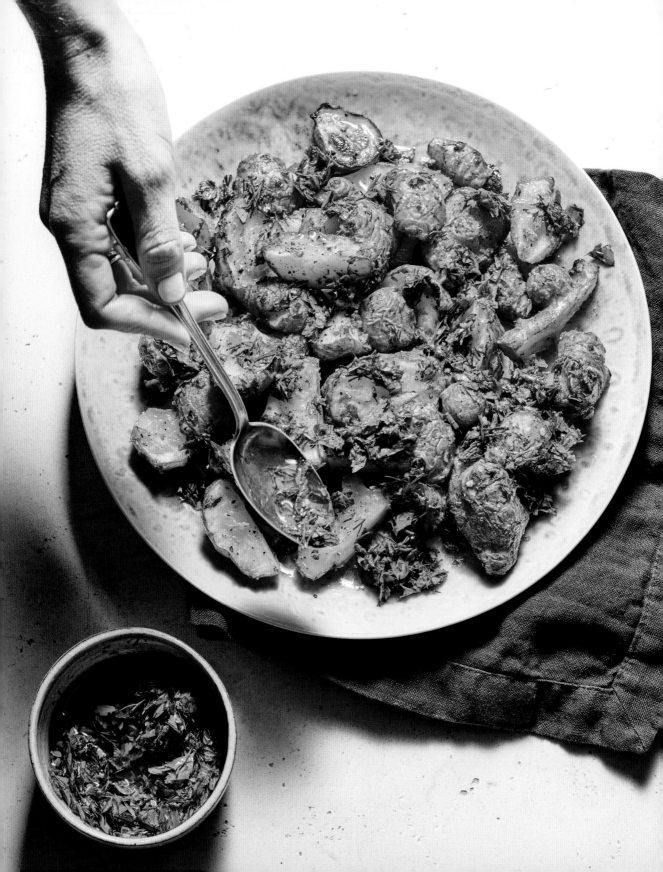

Roasted Sunchokes with Lotsa Herbs

Sunchokes are a great source of prebiotics (food for the good bacteria in your gut) you can get your hands on. Probiotic-rich food such as fermented foods and miso paste are critical for gut health, but it's important that we nourish our gut not only with these healthy microbes but also with the nutrients they need to flourish. Sunchokes are seasonal and can be found from fall until spring. If you're not able to find sunchokes at your local market or grocery store, you can make this recipe with baby potatoes or cauliflower florets.

SERVES 4

2 garlic cloves, chopped (about 2 teaspoons), divided

1 tablespoon Dijon mustard

¼ cup plus 2 tablespoons extra-virgin olive oil

1 pound sunchokes, cut in half lengthwise

Sea salt and freshly ground black pepper, to taste

½ cup chopped fresh parsley

¼ cup chopped fresh dill

¼ cup chopped fresh mint

½ tablespoon red pepper flakes

1 tablespoon champagne vinegar

Maldon sea salt, for serving

1. Preheat the oven to 400°F and line a baking sheet with parchment paper.

2. In a medium bowl, whisk together 1½ teaspoons of the garlic with the mustard and 2 tablespoons of the olive oil.

3. Add the sunchokes to the bowl and mix to combine. Season generously with salt and pepper.

4. On the prepared baking sheet, place the sunchokes cut side up and roast for 30 minutes, then broil for 2 to 3 minutes, checking every 30 seconds to make sure they don't burn.

5. While the sunchokes are roasting, make the dressing. In a small bowl, mix together the remaining ½ teaspoon of garlic with the parsley, dill, mint, red pepper flakes, champagne vinegar, and the remaining ¼ cup of the olive oil.

6. Transfer the sunchokes to a serving platter or bowl and top with the herb dressing and a sprinkle of Maldon sea salt.

Spicy Roasted Broccoli Rabe

A great side dish with a kick or meal-prep addition. Broccoli rabe is more tender than regular broccoli, which makes the stalks even more delicious to eat.

SERVES 4

1 pound broccoli rabe

2 tablespoons extra-virgin olive oil

½ tablespoon red pepper flakes

1 tablespoon lemon juice

Sea salt, to taste

1. Preheat the oven to 400°F.

2. In a large mixing bowl, combine the broccoli rabe, olive oil, red pepper flakes, lemon juice, and salt. Stir to coat the broccoli.

3. Arrange broccoli rabe evenly across one or two sheet pans, making sure not to overcrowd the pan.

4. Roast for 25 to 30 minutes, or until the edges look crisp but not burnt. Eat right away or store in an airtight container in the refrigerator for up to 5 days.

Turmeric Cauliflower

This dish was inspired by the prepared foods section at Erewhon in LA. I just could not get enough of this zesty, tangy cauliflower and decided to create my own version. I love having this alongside chicken or in the refrigerator for an addition to salads and grain bowls during the week.

SERVES 4

1 tablespoon julienned ginger

1 garlic clove, minced

½ teaspoon ground turmeric

¼ teaspoon ground cumin

¼ cup avocado oil

1 teaspoon lime zest

1 tablespoon lime juice, divided

3 cups cauliflower florets (from about 1 head)

Sea salt and freshly ground black pepper to taste

½ cup chopped fresh cilantro, stems included

1. Heat a large skillet over medium-high heat.

2. In a large mixing bowl, add the ginger, garlic, turmeric, cumin, avocado oil, lime zest, and ½ tablespoon of the lime juice, and whisk to combine.

3. Add the cauliflower to the ginger-garlic mixture and stir to coat completely. Season generously with salt and pepper.

4. Add the cauliflower to the preheated skillet and sauté, stirring occasionally, for 5 to 7 minutes, or until lightly brown.

5. Reduce the heat to medium, cover the skillet, and allow the cauliflower to steam for 5 minutes more, shaking the skillet every minute or so.

6. Remove the skillet from the heat, and add the remaining lime juice and the cilantro.

7. Store in an airtight container in the refrigerator for up to 5 days.

Purple Sweet Potato Fries

Purple sweet potatoes are a little denser and drier than regular sweet potatoes, which makes them perfect for French fries. Pair with the Minted Tahini Dip on page 192 for a delicious side dish or snack.

SERVES 4 TO 6

1 pound purple sweet potatoes (about 2 to 3 sweet potatoes)

2 tablespoons avocado oil

1 teaspoon ground cumin

1 teaspoon sea salt

1. Preheat the oven to 400°F.

2. Cut the sweet potatoes into ¼- to ½-inch-thick strips. The fries should be around 3 inches long, but it's okay if they vary in size.

3. In a large bowl, toss the sweet potatoes in the avocado oil and season with the cumin and sea salt.

4. On one or two baking sheets, spread the potatoes out, making sure not to overcrowd the pans. Bake for 30 to 35 minutes, flipping the sweet potatoes after 20 minutes.

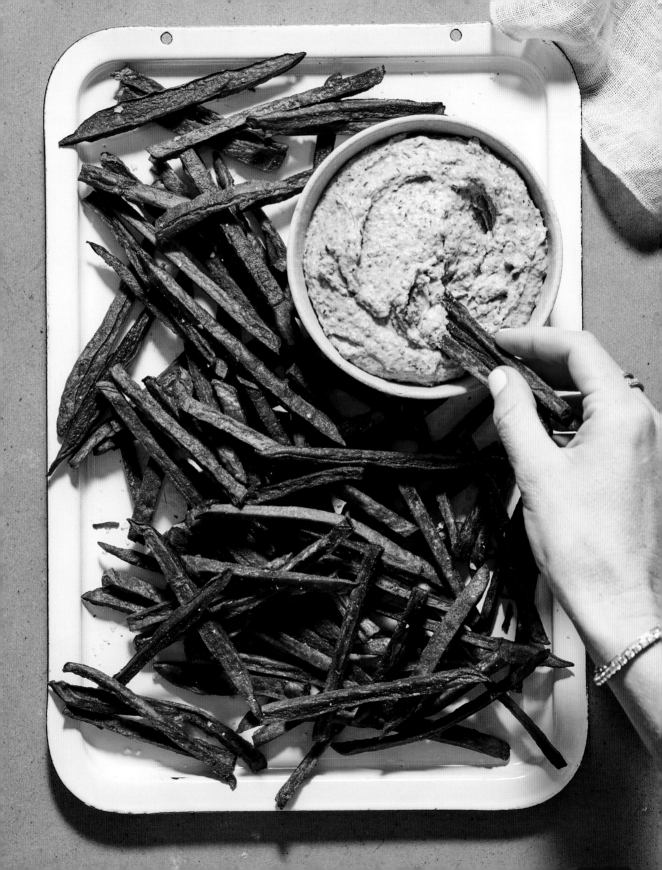

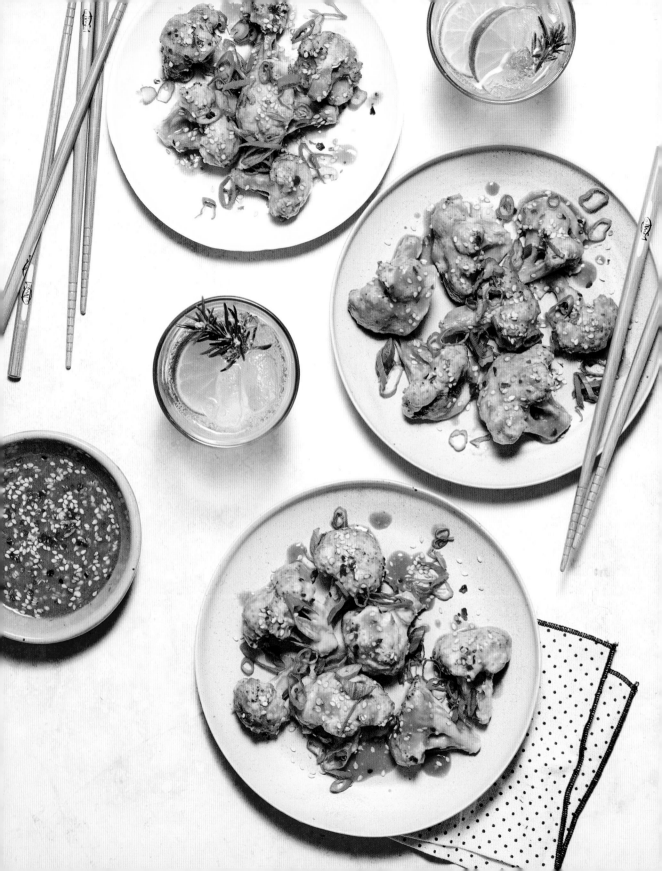

Sesame Broccoli Poppers

Broccoli is part of the cruciferous vegetable family, a class of vegetables that are excellent for detoxification liver support, and have anti-estrogen effects, which can reduce the risk of fibroids, polycystic ovary syndrome (PCOS), and some hormone-sensitive cancers.

SERVES 4 TO 6

1 cup gluten-free all-purpose flour (I like Bob's Redmill)

1 cup plus 1 tablespoon water

2 tablespoons sesame seeds, divided

3 cups broccoli florets (from about 1 head)

1 tablespoon white miso paste

1 tablespoon tamari

1 teaspoon lime juice

1 tablespoon coconut aminos

1 tablespoon toasted sesame oil

½ teaspoon red pepper flakes

Notes: This recipe works great in an air fryer as well! Reduce the heat to 370°F and cook for 4 to 5 minutes, toss in the sauce, and cook for an additional 4 to 5 minutes. Skip the broil at the end.

Feel free to double the sauce if you are making more than 3 cups of broccoli florets.

1. Preheat the oven to 400°F and line a baking sheet with parchment paper.

2. In a medium mixing bowl, whisk together the flour, 1 cup of the water, and 1 tablespoon of the sesame seeds.

3. Dip the broccoli florets in the flour mixture one by one, then place them on the prepared baking sheet. Bake the broccoli for 10 minutes.

4. While the broccoli is in the oven, in a medium mixing bowl, whisk together the white miso paste, the remaining tablespoon of water, and the tamari until combined. Add the lime juice, coconut aminos, sesame oil, red pepper flakes, and remaining sesame seeds.

5. Remove the broccoli from the oven and add to the bowl with the sauce, tossing until well combined. Return the broccoli to the baking sheet and bake for 10 minutes more.

6. Turn the oven to broil and broil for an additional 2 to 5 minutes, checking every minute to make sure the broccoli does not burn.

Spiced Carrot Salad

When I was a kid, my dad and I would go to this little deli on the water in Sausalito and we were obsessed with the carrot salad that came with our sandwiches—it was so simple and flavorful. We started making our own version of it at home, and here it is. A great side for barbeques or mezze-style meals.

SERVES 4

2 large carrots, peeled and shredded (about 4 cups)

1 tablespoon curry powder

2 tablespoons extra-virgin olive oil

2 tablespoons dried goji berries or currants

1 tablespoon toasted slivered almonds

¼ cup chopped fresh parsley

½ tablespoon Maldon sea salt

1. In a medium mixing bowl, add the carrots and curry powder, and toss to combine.

2. Add the olive oil, goji berries, slivered almonds, parsley, and sea salt, and mix thoroughly.

Warm Chicory Salad

Chicories are similar to lettuce, but heartier and a little bitter, so they stand up to heat really well and are perfect for winter salads. The addition of anchovies adds a salty, umami flavor, and a kick of anti-inflammatory omega-3 fatty acids. Anchovies are small fish, so they are a safe, low-mercury option as well. In the cooking process, the anchovies completely dissolve, making this dish suitable even for those who might be anchovy-hesitant.

SERVES 2 TO 4

¼ cup extra-virgin olive oil

1 medium shallot, diced

1 garlic clove, minced

4 anchovy fillets

1 tablespoon stone ground mustard

Juice of 1 lemon

2 heads chicory, leaves separated and torn (you can substitute radicchio, escarole, or a combination)

¼ cup toasted walnuts, roughly chopped

Maldon sea salt (for garnish)

Freshly ground black pepper (for garnish)

Shaved Pecorino cheese (for garnish) (optional)

1. In a large sauté pan, heat the olive oil over medium heat.

2. Add the shallot, garlic, and anchovies. Using a wooden spoon, stir and break up the anchovies until they dissolve into the olive oil and the shallots become translucent.

3. Stir in the mustard, then add the lemon juice.

4. Reduce heat to low, add the chicory leaves, and use tongs to thoroughly coat the leaves in the warm vinaigrette.

5. Plate and garnish with the toasted walnuts, a pinch of Maldon sea salt, pepper, and shaved Pecorino cheese, if using.

Hot & Cold Cucumber Salad

Cucumbers are a great vehicle for flavor; crunchy, fresh, and slightly bitter. I love seeing what chefs do with them, and will always order the cucumber salad off any menu I see it on. This version gets its flavor from toasted seeds, namely coriander. If this is your first time toasting whole coriander seeds, it certainly won't be the last!

SERVES 2 TO 4

2 tablespoons raw pumpkin seeds

1 tablespoon whole coriander seeds

½ tablespoon whole mustard seeds

4 Persian cucumbers

½ teaspoon Aleppo pepper or red pepper flakes

½ teaspoon sea salt

¼ cup parsley leaves, whole or torn

2 teaspoons champagne vinegar

1 tablespoon extra-virgin olive oil

1. In a medium frying pan over low heat, lightly toast the pumpkin, coriander, and mustard seeds. Cook, keeping an eye on the seeds and shaking the pan occasionally, until the seeds start to pop and become fragrant, 3 to 5 minutes.

2. While the seeds are toasting, cut the cucumbers in half lengthwise and then diagonally into 1-inch segments. Cut off and discard the ends.

3. In a medium mixing bowl, combine the cut cucumbers with the Aleppo pepper and sea salt.

4. Add the parsley leaves, champagne vinegar, and extra-virgin olive oil to the cucumbers. Toss to combine.

5. Add the toasted seeds and toss to coat with the vinaigrette.

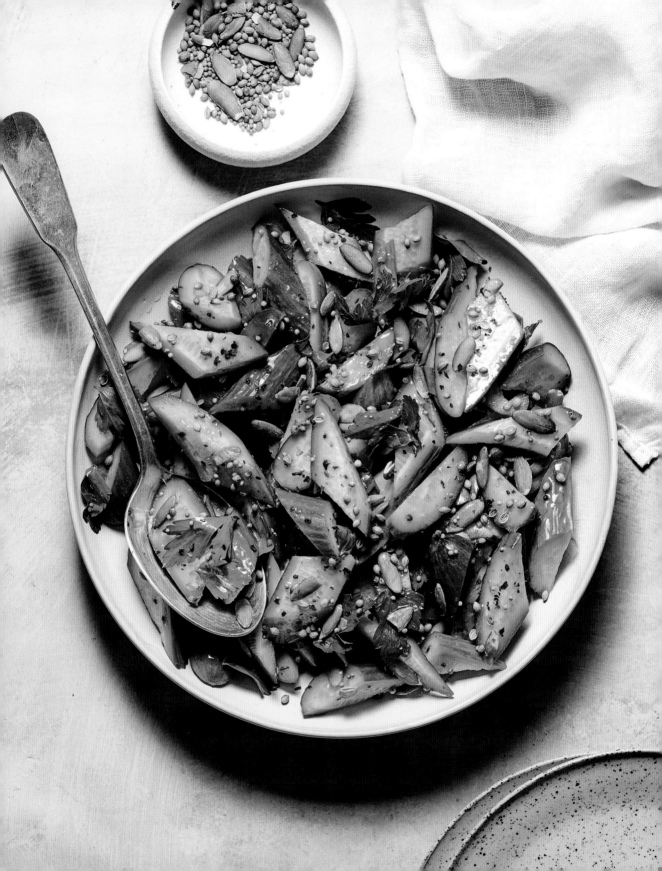

Simple Green Salad

A classic shallot vinaigrette is a culinary staple and is easy to whip up with ingredients you most likely already have in your pantry. I love how this salad is made entirely in the serving bowl; whisk the dressing together, throw the greens on top, and toss. Perfect for entertaining or simple weekday meals.

SERVES 2 TO 4

1 tablespoon finely chopped shallots

1 tablespoon red, white, or sherry vinegar

Pinch of sea salt

1 teaspoon Dijon mustard

4 tablespoons extra-virgin olive oil

4 to 6 cups mixed greens

½ cup fresh herbs, such as parsley, tarragon, and dill

Freshly ground black pepper (optional)

1. In a serving bowl, add the shallots, vinegar, and a pinch of salt. Whisk to combine and let the mixture sit for 5 to 10 minutes.

2. Whisk in the Dijon mustard and olive oil until fully emulsified.

3. Add the mixed greens to the serving bowl and toss to coat. Top with the fresh herbs and black pepper, if using.

Eggplant Caponata

This hearty eggplant caponata is a great complement to simply cooked meats and fish, and is delicious mixed in with gluten-free pasta and sautéed greens for a flavorful and plant-forward vegetarian meal. I love making this dish as part of a weekly meal prep— it's an easy way to incorporate variety into your weekly meals, and it is one of those dishes that just tastes better the next day.

SERVES 4 TO 6

1 eggplant, cut into ½-inch cubes

¼ cup extra-virgin olive oil, divided

Kosher salt and freshly ground black pepper, to taste

1 medium yellow onion, diced

2 garlic cloves, minced

1 bell pepper, deseeded and cut into ½-inch cubes

2 celery stalks, sliced ½-inch thick

2 tablespoons tomato paste

½ cup crushed tomatoes

2 tablespoons white wine or champagne vinegar

10 to 15 pitted green olives, quartered

2 tablespoons capers, drained

¼ cup raisins

¼ cup fresh basil leaves, chopped

¼ cup fresh parsley leaves, chopped

1. Preheat the oven to 375°F and line a baking sheet with parchment paper.

2. In a medium mixing bowl, combine the eggplant with 2 to 3 tablespoons of the olive oil, 1½ teaspoons of salt, and ½ teaspoon of pepper, stirring to coat the eggplant.

3. Place the eggplant on the prepared baking sheet and bake for 30 minutes, or until tender.

4. While the eggplant is baking, in a large skillet, heat the remaining olive oil over medium heat.

5. Add the onion, garlic, bell pepper, and celery, and sauté for 5 minutes, or until fragrant.

6. Add the tomato paste, and stir to combine. Add the crushed tomatoes, vinegar, olives, capers, and raisins. Reduce the heat to low, bring the mixture to a simmer, and season generously with salt and pepper.

7. Let the mixture simmer for at least 10 minutes, stirring occasionally, or until the eggplant is done cooking.

8. Remove the eggplant from the oven and add it to the pan with the rest of the vegetables. Stir to combine and allow the vegetable mixture to cook for 5 minutes more.

9. Stir the basil and parsley into the caponata and season with additional salt and pepper to taste.

VEGETABLES & SALADS

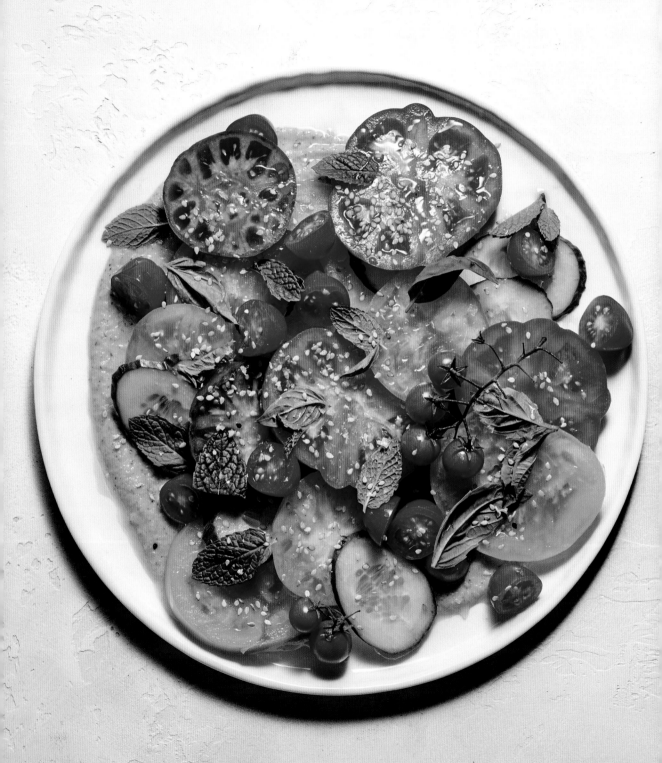

Heirloom Tomato, Sesame & Herb Salad with Green Miso Dressing

Tomatoes need little intervention during peak season, and I love how this dish accentuates the freshness of ripe heirloom tomatoes, while offering a new twist on our usual (but always delicious) tomato and basil preparation.

SERVES 2 TO 4

½ **medium zucchini, roughly chopped**

1 **tablespoon white miso paste**

Zest and juice of 1 lime

¼ **cup plus 1 tablespoon extra-virgin olive oil**

1½ **tablespoons rice wine vinegar, divided**

3 **heirloom tomatoes**

3 **to 5 cherry tomatoes**

1 **medium cucumber (see Note)**

5 **to 7 fresh basil leaves**

3 **to 5 fresh mint leaves**

2 **to 3 tablespoons gomasio (see Note)**

Notes: Lemon cucumbers are fantastic here, but can be hard to find, so any cucumber will work.

Gomasio is a Japanese sesame seed and salt blend. It's fantastic, and I highly recommend keeping a bottle in your pantry, but if you don't have gomasio, you can substitute white sesame seeds and sea salt.

1. Start by making the dressing. In a blender or food processor, add the zucchini, miso paste, lime zest and juice, ¼ cup of the olive oil, and 1 tablespoon of the rice wine vinegar, and blend until smooth. The dressing can be made up to 3 days in advance and kept in the refrigerator.

2. Slice the tomatoes and cucumber into rounds and place in a bowl. (I like to use different-colored tomatoes when available.) Dress the tomatoes and cucumbers with the remaining tablespoon of the olive oil and ½ tablespoon of the rice wine vinegar.

3. When ready to serve, spread a generous layer of the dressing over the bottom of a large plate. Arrange the tomatoes, cucumbers, basil leaves, and mint leaves on top of the dressing. Top with a generous sprinkle of gomasio.

Quinoa & Arugula Salad

Make a batch of quinoa during your weekly meal prep so you can throw this salad together in minutes. It's hearty, satisfying, and a great vehicle for your favorite protein.

SERVES 4

1 tablespoon diced shallot

Juice of 1 lemon

Sea salt

1 tablespoon whole grain
   mustard

¼ cup extra-virgin olive oil

3 cups arugula

1 cup quinoa, cooked
   and cooled to room
   temperature

½ cup toasted walnuts

1 cup fresh parsley leaves,
   roughly chopped

Freshly ground black pepper,
   to taste

1. Start by making the dressing. In a serving bowl, combine the shallot, lemon juice, and a pinch of salt. Let the mixture sit for 3 to 5 minutes.

2. Whisk in the mustard, then slowly pour in the olive oil, whisking until the dressing emulsifies.

3. Add the arugula, quinoa, walnuts, and parsley to the bowl, and toss. Finish with a generous pinch of salt and pepper.

Meal-Prep Roasted Vegetables

An every-week kind of dish, this vegetable medley is great alongside your favorite protein, in a gluten-free pasta, or on a salad, and simply having these vegetables prepped and in the refrigerator will increase your vegetable consumption and make weekday meals much easier to throw together.

SERVES 4

2 cups mixed mushrooms, quartered

1 zucchini, sliced 1-inch thick

1 yellow squash, sliced 1-inch thick

1 red onion, diced

1 red bell pepper, sliced 1-inch thick

5 celery stalks, sliced ¼-inch thick

⅓ cup extra-virgin olive oil

2 teaspoons sea salt

Leaves from 5 to 10 fresh thyme sprigs

¼ cup fresh basil, chopped

¼ cup fresh parsley, chopped

1. Preheat the oven to 375°F and line a baking sheet with parchment paper.

2. In a mixing bowl, combine the mushrooms, zucchini, squash, onion, bell pepper, celery, olive oil, salt, and thyme leaves. Stir to combine.

3. Spread the vegetable mixture evenly across the prepared baking sheet and bake for 30 to 40 minutes, or until the vegetables are lightly browned.

4. Remove the vegetables from the oven and top with the basil and parsley. Serve immediately or store in an airtight container in the refrigerator for up to 5 days.

VEGETABLES & SALADS

Rainbow Chop with Carrot-Ginger Dressing

This salad is incredibly versatile. Make extra dressing, as you will want to put this on everything; it goes great with grilled shrimp, chicken, fish, and avocado as well!

SERVES 4

¼ cup carrots, peeled and sliced into large chunks

¼ cup cashews, soaked overnight

1 tablespoon apple cider vinegar

3 tablespoons extra-virgin olive oil, divided

1 thumb-size piece ginger

Sea salt, to taste

1 to 2 tablespoons water, divided

2 heads romaine lettuce, washed and chopped

1 head radicchio, washed and chopped

¼ cup scallions, green and white parts, sliced ¼-inch thick

½ medium avocado, peeled and pit removed, sliced

1 tablespoon sesame seeds

1. Start by making the dressing. In a food processor, add the carrots, cashews, apple cider vinegar, 2 tablespoons of the olive oil, ginger, ½ teaspoon of the salt, and 1 tablespoon of the water, and pulse until smooth. It may take a while to get the cashews, carrots, and ginger to blend completely, so be patient!

2. Season the dressing with salt to taste, and, if it's too thick, add more water as necessary, 1 tablespoon at a time. The dressing can be made 1 to 2 days in advance.

3. In a serving bowl, add the romaine, radicchio, and scallions. Dress the greens with the remaining tablespoon of olive oil and season with a pinch of salt.

4. Spoon the carrot-ginger dressing on top and toss to combine. Top with the sliced avocado and sesame seeds and serve alongside your favorite protein.

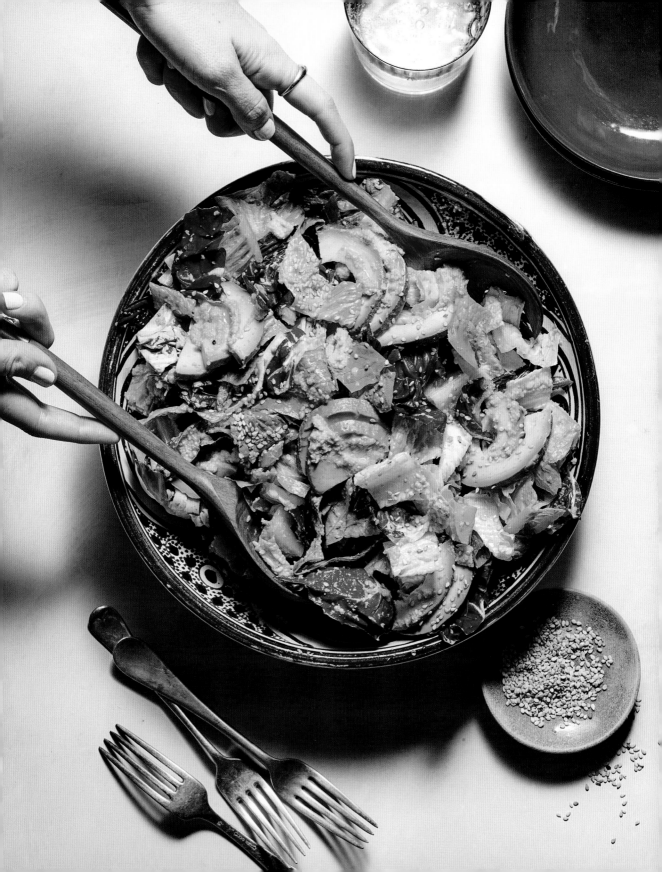

Mixed Green Salad with Ginger, Carrots & Mulberries

This salad is light, sweet, and crunchy at all once. It's just as satisfying as a simple lunch alongside your favorite protein as it is at a barbeque shared among friends. I particularly love the dried mulberries in here; they are slightly sweet and chewy, adding great texture and flavor to this salad.

SERVES 4

Juice of 1 lemon

2 teaspoons coconut aminos

1 teaspoon grated ginger

¼ cup extra-virgin olive oil

¼ cup raw almonds, toasted and chopped

Sea salt

4 to 6 cups mixed greens

⅓ cup carrots, julienned

½ cup microgreens

¼ cup dried mulberries

6 to 10 fresh mint leaves, torn and roughly chopped

Freshly ground black pepper, to taste

1. Start by making the dressing. In a small bowl, whisk together the lemon juice and coconut aminos. Add the ginger, then slowly whisk in the olive oil. Add the chopped almonds and a pinch of sea salt, and set aside.

2. In a medium bowl, combine the mixed greens, carrots, microgreens, dried mulberries, and mint leaves.

3. When ready to serve, dress the salad and season with a pinch of sea salt and black pepper.

Celery, Fennel & Apple Salad

Celery is underrated; incredibly crunchy, hydrating, and fresh, it makes the perfect pairing for hearty fennel and tart apple slices. The mustard vinaigrette ties it all together to make a flavorful and satisfying salad.

SERVES 4

½ tablespoon whole grain mustard

1 tablespoon apple cider vinegar

2 tablespoons extra-virgin olive oil

Sea salt and freshly ground black pepper, to taste

¼ cup toasted almonds, roughly chopped

1 fennel bulb, sliced thin with a mandoline (reserve the fronds if possible)

4 celery stalks, sliced ¼-inch thick

1 medium tart apple, such as Gala, Fuji, or Pink Lady, quartered and thinly sliced

1. In a medium mixing bowl, add the mustard and apple cider vinegar, and whisk to combine.

2. Slowly whisk in the olive oil. Season with salt and pepper to taste, then mix in the almonds and stir to combine.

3. Add the sliced fennel bulb and fronds (if using), celery, and apple. Toss to thoroughly coat with the dressing, then taste to check the seasoning.

Noodles
& Grains

Lemongrass Black Rice

Black rice gets its signature black-purple hue from anthocyanin, a potent antioxidant also found in blueberries, blackberries, and cherries. Make sure not to skip the soaking step, or those wonderful anthocyanins might stain your teeth!

SERVES 6 TO 8

2 cups black rice

2 tablespoons avocado oil

1 shallot, diced (about ¼ cup)

1-inch piece ginger, diced

1 garlic clove, minced

½ lemongrass stalk, cut lengthwise, or ½ teaspoon ground lemongrass

1 whole star anise

1 bay leaf

2 cups full-fat unsweetened coconut milk

2 cups chicken or vegetable broth

Sea salt to taste

Sliced scallions (for garnish)

Crispy Shallots (page 215) (for garnish)

1. Soak the black rice in cold water for at least 4 hours or up to overnight.

2. In a medium saucepan, heat the avocado oil over medium heat. Add the shallot, ginger, and garlic, and stir until fragrant.

3. Add the lemongrass, star anise, and bay leaf, followed by the rice, coconut milk, and broth. Season generously with salt.

4. Bring the mixture to a boil, then reduce heat to a simmer and cook for 30 minutes, or until all the liquid has been absorbed. Fluff with a fork and serve topped with sliced scallions and crispy shallots.

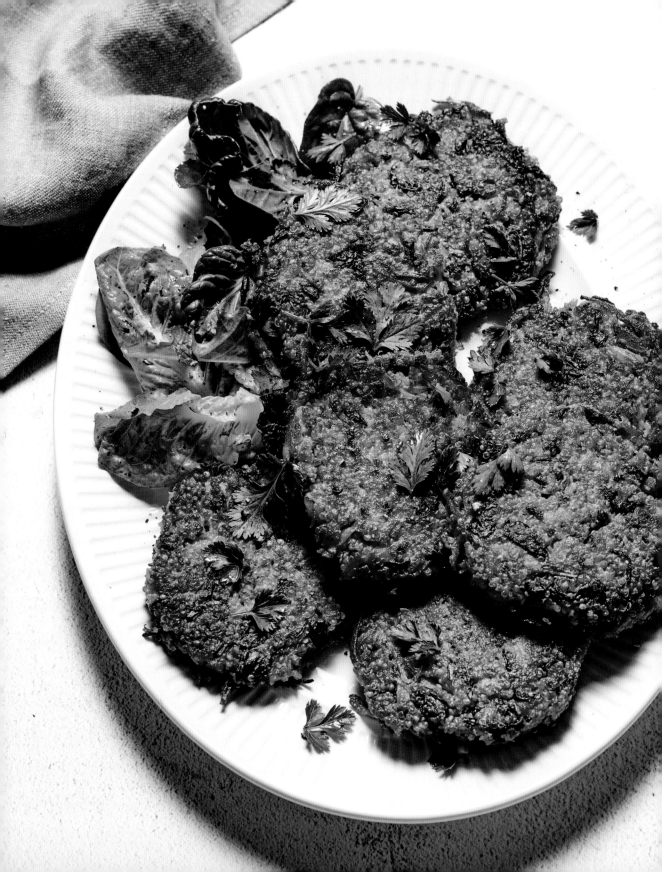

Spiced Quinoa Cakes

Full of protein, fiber-rich vegetables and quinoa, healthy fats, and nourishing spices, these cakes are great for vegetarians and are the perfect topping for salads and sautéed greens, or as a snack.

MAKES ABOUT 15 CAKES

1 cup uncooked quinoa

¼ to ½ cup extra-virgin olive oil, plus more as needed

1 small yellow onion, diced

2 garlic cloves, minced

1-inch piece ginger, peeled and diced

1 medium carrot, peeled and shredded

1 small sweet potato, peeled and shredded (about 1 cup)

¼ cup chopped fresh cilantro

1 cup spinach, roughly chopped

1 teaspoon ground cumin

½ teaspoon ground coriander

¼ teaspoon ground turmeric

⅛ teaspoon smoked paprika

Sea salt and freshly ground black pepper, to taste

2 large eggs

1. Cook the quinoa according to package directions.

2. While the quinoa is cooking, prepare the vegetables. In a medium skillet, heat 2 tablespoons of the olive oil over medium heat. Add the onion, garlic, and ginger, and stir until fragrant, 2 to 3 minutes.

3. Add the shredded carrot and sweet potato. Cook, stirring occasionally, for 5 minutes more. Add the cilantro and spinach, and cook for another 2 to 3 minutes, or until the spinach has wilted.

4. In a mixing bowl, combine the cooked quinoa and vegetables and season with the cumin, coriander, turmeric, paprika, salt, and pepper. Taste, adjust seasoning, and allow the mixture to cool.

5. In a separate bowl, whisk the eggs together, then add the eggs to the quinoa mixture.

6. In a medium to large skillet, heat 2 tablespoons of the olive oil over medium heat. Use a measuring cup to portion ¼ cup of the quinoa mixture and form it into a disc using your hands.

7. Pan-fry the quinoa cakes for 2 to 3 minutes on each side, or until lightly browned. Continue until all the mixture has been used, adding more olive oil to the skillet as needed.

Socca Flatbread

Socca is a traditional dish popular in Italy and the South of France. Made with chickpea flour, socca is high in protein and fiber and is gluten free! Top with tomato sauce and basil to make a pizza, or serve alongside a salad and your favorite protein.

SERVES 2 TO 4

1 cup chickpea flour

1 cup warm water

1 tablespoon extra-virgin olive oil, plus more for greasing the pan

2 tablespoons fresh herbs (such as basil, parsley, and dill)

½ teaspoon sea salt

¼ teaspoon freshly ground black pepper

1. In a medium bowl, whisk together the chickpea flour, water, olive oil, herbs, sea salt, and pepper. Let the mixture sit for at least 30 minutes, or up to 12 hours.

2. Preheat the oven to 425°F and place a 12-inch cast-iron skillet in the oven as it preheats.

3. Take the cast-iron skillet out of the oven and grease generously with olive oil.

4. Pour the socca batter into the hot skillet and cook for 15 minutes. Serve immediately.

Herbed Brown Rice & Cauliflower Pilaf

Cauliflower rice is fooling no one. There is nothing like actual rice, but in this dish, I find the cauliflower adds extra texture and flavor, while cutting the carbohydrate count in half and increasing your vegetable intake. If you are using fresh cauliflower, you can make cauliflower rice by pulsing the cauliflower in a food processor, but frozen cauliflower rice is also perfectly acceptable and very easy.

SERVES 2

½ cup long-grain brown rice

1 tablespoon extra-virgin olive oil

1 medium shallot, minced

1 cup chicken or vegetable broth

2 cups cauliflower rice (fresh or frozen)

¼ cup chopped fresh parsley

1 teaspoon lemon zest

1 tablespoon lemon juice (see Note)

Sea salt and freshly ground black pepper, to taste

Note: If you have preserved lemon, you can swap the lemon zest and juice for 1 tablespoon of diced preserved lemon peel.

1. Rinse the brown rice until the liquid is clear or slightly hazy and set aside.

2. In a medium saucepan, heat the olive oil over medium heat. Add the shallot, and cook until translucent, 3 to 5 minutes.

3. Add the brown rice to the saucepan, and toast until fragrant, 2 to 3 minutes. Add the broth and a generous pinch of sea salt, and bring to a boil.

4. Reduce the heat to a simmer and cook, covered, for 35 to 40 minutes, or until about 90 percent of the liquid has been absorbed.

5. Stir in the cauliflower rice, and heat until the cauliflower rice is cooked through and all the liquid has evaporated. Add in the parsley, lemon zest, and lemon juice, and stir to combine.

6. Season with sea salt and pepper as desired.

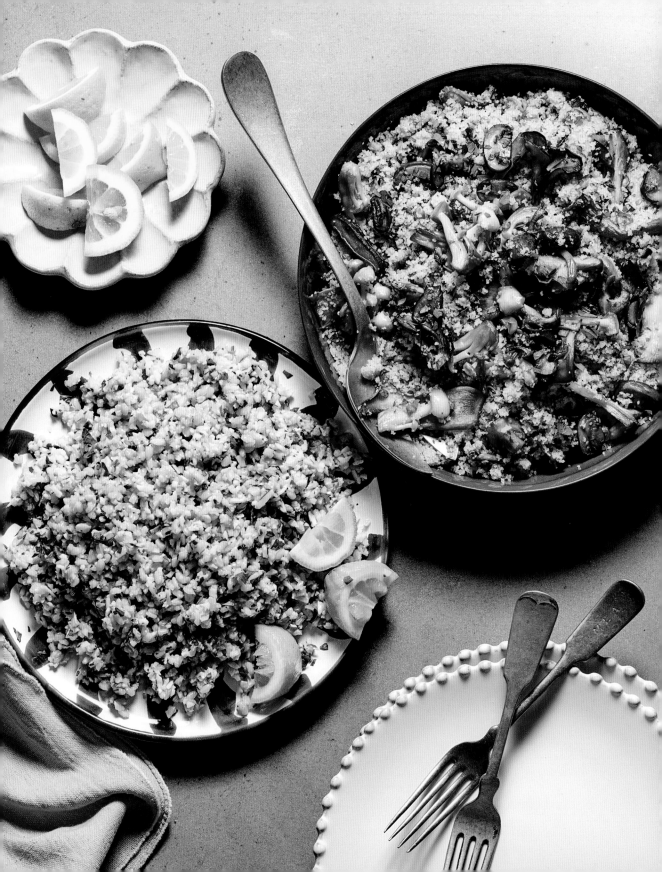

Mushrooms & Fonio

Fonio is an ancient grain of African heritage that is consumed widely in West African countries. It's naturally gluten-free and fiber-rich, and it's a great source of B vitamins. I love it as an alternative to couscous. Make this dish a meal by adding some sautéed greens and a couple runny eggs. If you can't find fonio, use quinoa instead, which is also fiber and protein rich.

SERVES 4

1 tablespoon extra-virgin olive oil, divided

½ tablespoon ghee

4 to 6 cups mixed mushrooms (at least three different varieties), roughly chopped

Sea salt

1 medium shallot, diced

1 garlic clove, minced

Leaves from 2 sprigs fresh thyme

1 teaspoon lime zest

1 tablespoon lime juice

1 cup fonio

2 cups chicken or vegetable broth

Freshly ground black pepper, to taste

1 cup chopped fresh parsley

1. In a large skillet, heat ½ tablespoon of the olive oil and the ghee over medium-high heat.

2. Add the mushrooms, and season generously with salt. Stir until the mushrooms decrease in size by roughly one quarter, then add the shallot and garlic.

3. Add the thyme, lime zest, and lime juice. Reduce the heat to medium and cook, stirring frequently, until mushrooms are cooked down by half, 5 to 10 minutes.

4. In a medium pot, add the fonio and the remaining ½ tablespoon olive oil, and increase the heat to medium. Stir to combine, then add the broth. Bring to a boil, then reduce the heat and let simmer, covered, for 1 minute. Turn off the heat and let it steam for 5 minutes.

5. Fluff the fonio with a fork and season with salt and pepper. Add the mushroom mixture and parsley to the fonio and stir to combine.

Super Green Spaghetti with Zucchini Pesto

I was very anti-zoodle until I started making this recipe, which has become a weekly staple in my house. This dish takes less than thirty minutes to make, and everyone in my family enjoys it, despite the fact that half the noodles are actually zucchini.

SERVES 4

4 ounces gluten-free spaghetti noodles (I like Banza)

1 medium zucchini, roughly chopped, plus 2 medium zucchinis, spiralized

1 whole garlic clove, plus 1 garlic clove, minced

¼ cup plus 1 tablespoon extra-virgin olive oil

Juice of 1 lemon

½ cup fresh basil leaves

¼ cup pine nuts, toasted

Sea salt and freshly ground black pepper, to taste

1. Bring a large pot of salted water to a boil. Cook the noodles according to package instructions. Drain and set aside.

2. Meanwhile, make the pesto. In a blender, combine the zucchini, whole garlic clove, ¼ cup of the olive oil, lemon juice, basil leaves, and pine nuts. Blend until smooth, and season with salt and pepper to taste.

3. In a large skillet, heat the remaining tablespoon of olive oil over medium heat.

4. Add the minced garlic to the pan and stir for 1 minute, or until fragrant but not brown.

5. Add the spiralized zucchini. Toss the mixture with tongs until the zucchini noodles start to cook but don't fall apart, 3 to 5 minutes.

6. Add the cooked spaghetti and the zucchini pesto, and stir to combine.

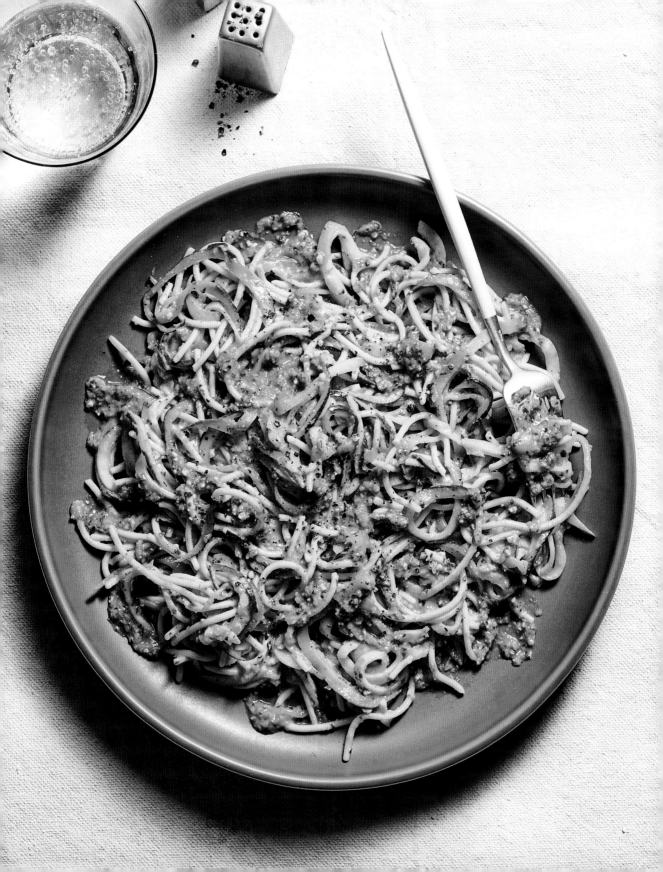

Chicken, Peanut & Soba Noodle Salad

Soba noodles are traditionally made from buckwheat, which has no relation to classic wheat, the primary source of gluten. Make sure to buy gluten-free soba noodles, as some might have a bit of whole wheat flour in them. Be careful not to overcook your noodles, or they will deteriorate.

SERVES 4 TO 6

1 lemon, sliced

1 bay leaf

2 boneless, skinless chicken breasts

1 (10-ounce) package gluten-free soba noodles

¼ cup smooth peanut butter

¼ cup toasted sesame oil

2 tablespoons rice wine vinegar

¼ cup filtered water

2 tablespoons coconut aminos

½ garlic clove

2 to 3 medium carrots, peeled and shredded (about 1 cup)

½ head cabbage, shredded (about 4 cups)

3 scallions, both white and green parts, thinly sliced (about ⅓ cup)

½ cup cilantro, chopped (stems included)

1 fresh Thai chili or cayenne pepper, deseeded and sliced (optional)

Sea salt, to taste

¼ cup sesame seeds, toasted

¼ cup dry roasted peanuts, roughly chopped

1. In a large pot, bring 8 cups of heavily salted water to a boil. Add the lemon slices and bay leaf, then add the chicken.

2. Bring to a boil and turn off the heat. Allow to cook for at least 20 minutes, but up to 1 hour.

3. Remove the chicken from the water, allow to cool, then shred with two forks and set aside.

4. While the chicken is cooking, cook the soba noodles according to package directions. Drain and run cold water over the cooked noodles to stop the cooking process.

5. To make the dressing, in a blender, combine the peanut butter, sesame oil, rice wine vinegar, water, coconut aminos, and garlic, and blend until smooth and creamy. (A hand blender also works well for this.)

6. In a large bowl, combine the carrots, cabbage, scallions, cilantro, Thai chili, soba noodles, and shredded chicken. Toss to combine and season lightly with salt.

7. Add the dressing and stir to coat, then add the sesame seeds and peanuts. Serve cool.

Fusilli with Braised Chicken Thighs, Mushrooms, Spinach & Sun-Dried Tomato Pesto

The key to this pasta is the ratio; there's more chicken and vegetables than pasta. It feels just as hearty and comforting as a big bowl of pasta, but with less blood sugar–spiking carbohydrates.

SERVES 2 TO 4

6 sun-dried tomatoes, drained

1 cup fresh basil

1 garlic clove

¼ cup toasted pine nuts

¼ cup plus 2 tablespoons extra-virgin olive oil

2 tablespoons lemon juice, divided

Sea salt and freshly ground black pepper, to taste

1 pound boneless, skinless chicken thighs

1 cup chicken stock

4 ounces gluten-free fusilli

15 to 20 button mushrooms, quartered

4 cups spinach

Red pepper flakes (for serving)

1. Make the sun-dried tomato pesto. In a food processor, combine the sun-dried tomatoes, basil, garlic, pine nuts, ¼ cup of the olive oil, and 1 tablespoon of the lemon juice, and pulse until combined. Season with salt and pepper and set aside.

2. In a large skillet, heat 1 tablespoon of the olive oil over high heat.

3. Generously season the chicken thighs with salt and pepper, then add the chicken, flesh side down, to the hot pan.

4. Cook the chicken until brown, about 3 minutes on one side, then flip and brown the other side, about 3 minutes more.

5. To the skillet, add the chicken broth and bring to a boil. Reduce the heat to a simmer and cook until the liquid evaporates, 5 to 10 minutes.

6. While the chicken is braising, cook the pasta according to the package instructions. Drain and set aside.

7. Remove the chicken from the pan and let it cool.

8. In the same skillet over high heat, deglaze with the remaining tablespoon of lemon juice. Add the remaining tablespoon of olive oil, then the mushrooms.

9. Season the pan sauce with sea salt and stir continuously for about 3 minutes, then reduce the heat to a simmer. Add the spinach, and stir occasionally until wilted.

10. Using two forks, shred the chicken into bite-size pieces. Add the chicken to the skillet, followed by the pasta and the sun-dried tomato pesto.

11. Stir the pesto to coat the pasta and serve with a sprinkle of sea salt and some red pepper flakes.

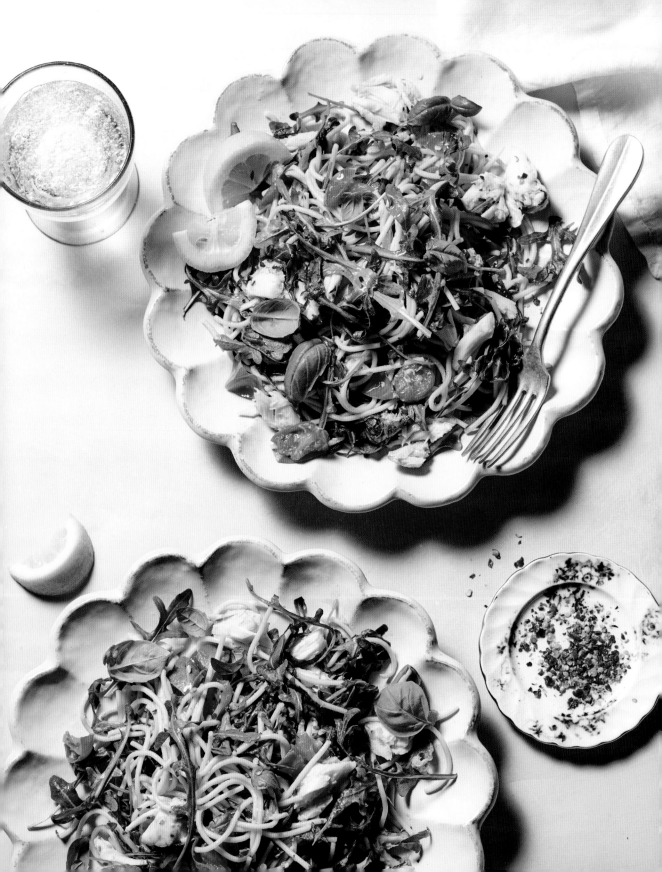

Fresh Crab & Arugula Spaghetti

Easy to throw together and impressively delicious, this is the type of dish you could whip up on a Tuesday night or make when your friends come over for dinner. This dish is best with fresh crab meat. Go to your local seafood market and see if they have freshly cracked crab, or if you're feeling ambitious you could crack the crab yourself!

SERVES 4

2 tablespoons extra-virgin olive oil

1 shallot, diced

2 garlic cloves, thinly sliced

½ to 1 tablespoon red pepper flakes (depending on the level of spice you like)

1 teaspoon oregano, dried or chopped fresh

1 cup cherry tomatoes, quartered

½ cup chicken or vegetable stock

Zest and juice of 1 lemon

Sea salt and freshly ground black pepper, to taste

8 ounces gluten-free spaghetti

1 pound fresh crab meat

4 cups arugula

Fresh basil leaves (for serving)

1. In a large skillet, heat the olive oil over medium heat. Add the shallot and garlic, and sauté, stirring frequently, until fragrant, about 2 minutes.

2. Add the red pepper flakes, oregano, and cherry tomatoes, and stir to combine. Sauté for 2 minutes more.

3. Add the chicken stock and lemon juice, and reduce the heat to a simmer. Cook until the sauce thickens, about 10 minutes. Season with salt and pepper to taste.

4. While the sauce is simmering, cook the pasta according to the package directions. Drain the pasta, reserving ¼ cup of the pasta water to add to the sauce.

5. Add the pasta to the skillet, using tongs to evenly incorporate. Add some of the reserved pasta water to adjust the sauce consistency, as needed.

6. Portion and serve with basil leaves, and an additional seasoning of salt and pepper if desired.

Shrimp & Veggie Pad Thai

The trick to succulent shrimp is not overcooking them. Shrimp cook quick, so make sure your pan is hot, that your shrimp are all roughly the same size, and do not overly crowd the shrimp in the pan. This will ensure they're all done at the same time.

SERVES 4

FOR THE SHRIMP
1 thumb-size piece ginger, julienned

1 garlic clove, minced

½ teaspoon ground turmeric

½ teaspoon ground cumin

½ teaspoon ground coriander

2 tablespoons avocado oil

1 pound jumbo wild shrimp, peeled and deveined

Sea salt to taste

1 lime, halved

FOR THE PAD THAI
1 (12-ounce) package brown rice pad Thai noodles

1 medium yellow squash

2 medium zucchinis

1 medium carrot, peeled

1 medium red bell pepper

¼ cup fresh cilantro, roughly chopped

¼ cup fresh mint, roughly chopped

¼ cup fresh basil, roughly chopped

1 tablespoon sesame seeds

2 tablespoons scallions, sliced

FOR THE DRESSING
¼ cup sunflower seed butter

¼ cup tablespoon tamari

¼ cup apple cider vinegar

¼ cup sesame oil

2 teaspoons fish sauce

Juice of 1 lime

¼ cup water

½ teaspoon fresh garlic, grated with a Microplane

½ teaspoon fresh ginger, grated with a Microplane

Note: If making this for meal prep, keep the dressing, salad, and shrimp separate. The shrimp will keep for 3 days in the refrigerator, and the salad and dressing will last 5 days.

1. Marinate the shrimp. In a bowl, combine the ginger, garlic, turmeric, cumin, coriander and avocado oil, and whisk to combine. Add the shrimp and a generous pinch of salt and stir to coat. Let sit for 15 to 30 minutes.

2. While the shrimp is marinating, cook the noodles according to package directions, then drain and rinse with cold water.

3. Use a mandoline to cut the yellow squash, zucchini, carrot, and bell pepper into thin strips about the same size as the noodles. You can also use a spiralizer, but you'll need to deseed and cut the bell pepper into thin slices with a knife.

4. In a large bowl, combine the vegetables and cooked noodles, toss, and set aside.

5. Make the dressing. In a bowl, combine the sunflower seed butter, tamari, apple cider vinegar, sesame oil, fish sauce, lime juice, water, garlic, and ginger. Whisk together until creamy. The dressing may thicken as it sets, so feel free to add some water, 1 tablespoon at a time, until it reaches the desired consistency.

6. Heat a large saucepan over high heat, then add the shrimp with the marinade. Reduce the heat to medium-high and stir until the shrimp are pink and cooked through, 3 to 4 minutes. Squeeze some lime juice over the shrimp and remove from the pan to prevent the shrimp from overcooking.

7. To serve, mix the dressing with the noodles and vegetables to fully combine.

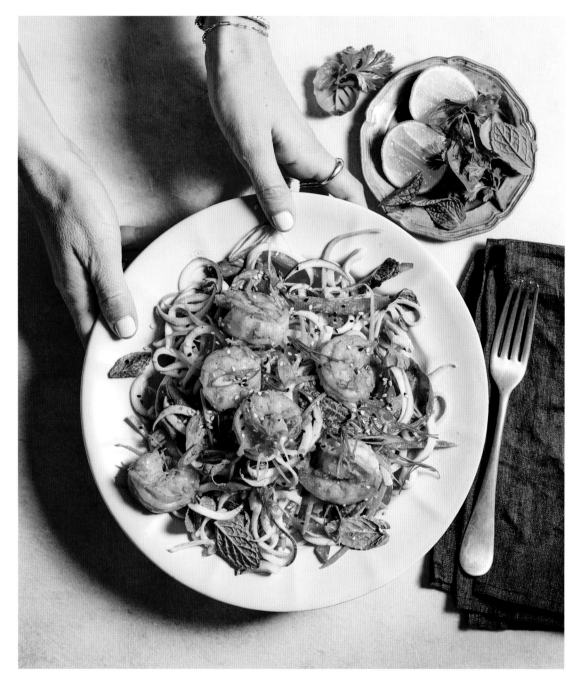

8. Add the cilantro, mint, basil, and sesame seeds, plus ¾ of the scallions, leaving a few for garnish.

9. Portion the pad Thai equally into four bowls and top with 5 to 6 shrimp, depending on the size.

10. Garnish with the leftover scallions and serve.

Meat, Poultry & Seafood

Chimichurri Steak Salad with Chickpea Croutons

In this dish, a classic chimichurri marinade for the steak doubles as the salad dressing. This herbaceous, zesty, and slightly spicy blend is a staple in Argentinian cuisine. It is similar to pesto, but has a parsley and vinegar base, instead of basil and lemon. Make sure to dress all components of this salad individually so you get a tangy hit of chimichurri in each bite.

SERVES 3 TO 4

1 shallot, minced

1 garlic clove, minced

1 teaspoon red pepper flakes

¼ cup red wine vinegar

½ teaspoon Maldon sea salt, plus more as needed

¼ cup fresh cilantro, finely chopped

¼ cup fresh parsley, finely chopped

2 tablespoons fresh oregano, finely chopped

Zest and juice of 1 lemon

½ cup plus 1½ tablespoons extra-virgin olive oil

1 to 1½ pounds skirt steak

2 cups sugar snap peas

4 cups mixed greens

2 medium tomatoes, quartered

¼ cup Pickled Red Onions (page 210) (for serving)

Crispy Smoked Paprika Chickpeas (page 194) (for serving)

Freshly ground black pepper, to taste

1. Make the chimichurri dressing. In a bowl, combine the shallot, garlic, red pepper flakes, red wine vinegar, and ½ teaspoon sea salt. Let the mixture sit for at least 5 minutes.

2. Add the cilantro, parsley, oregano, and lemon zest to the bowl, then whisk in ½ cup of the olive oil.

3. Marinate the steak with ½ half of the chimichurri dressing for at least 30 minutes before grilling.

4. Heat a frying pan over medium-high heat. Add a tablespoon of the olive oil, followed by the snap peas.

5. Squeeze half of the lemon juice over the snap peas, and sauté until blistered, about 3 to 5 minutes. Season with salt and set aside to cool.

6. Heat the grill or a grill pan over high heat. Add the marinated steak, and cook for 3 to 5 minutes on each side, or until clear grill lines appear. Set the steak aside to rest for at least 5 minutes, then slice the steak against the grain into 1-inch-thick slices.

7. In a large bowl, add the mixed greens and dress with the remaining olive oil and lemon juice. Season with salt.

8. To serve, portion in individual bowls or family-style on a platter. Divide the plate or bowl into quarters. Pile the dressed lettuce in one quarter, followed by the blistered snap peas, tomatoes, and steak. Drizzle the chimichurri over the salad, then top with pickled onions, crispy chickpeas, and pepper to taste.

Turkey Lettuce Wraps

P.F. Chang's lettuce wraps are nothing short of legendary. Luckily, they're also surprisingly quick and easy to replicate at home. This recipe features a savory turkey filling inside crispy lettuce cups that are topped with fresh pickled carrots.

SERVES 2 TO 4

FOR THE QUICK PICKLED CARROTS
1 medium carrot, julienned

¼ cup rice wine vinegar

Pinch of sea salt

FOR THE SAUCE
3 tablespoons gluten-free tamari

1½ tablespoons smooth peanut butter

2 tablespoons fresh lime juice

1 tablespoon toasted sesame oil

½ tablespoon grated ginger

1 teaspoon grated garlic

FOR THE TURKEY FILLING
2 tablespoons avocado oil, divided

1 pound ground turkey

Sea salt, to taste

1 medium shallot, diced

1 thumb-size piece ginger, peeled and thinly sliced

1 garlic clove, finely chopped

7 to 10 cremini or button mushrooms, finely chopped

¼ cup water chestnuts, finely chopped

½ cup toasted cashews, chopped

½ cup plus 1 tablespoon scallions, thinly sliced

FOR ASSEMBLY
1 head butter lettuce, leaves washed and separated

Cilantro leaves, for garnish

1. Make the quick-pickled carrots. In a shallow bowl, combine the julienned carrot with the rice wine vinegar and sea salt. Set aside for at least 30 minutes.

2. Make the sauce. In a medium bowl, whisk together the tamari, peanut butter, lime juice, sesame oil, ginger, and garlic.

3. Heat a cast-iron skillet or wok over medium-high heat and add 1 tablespoon of the avocado oil. Add the ground turkey and season generously with sea salt. Cook, breaking up the ground turkey with a wooden spoon, until it is browned and slightly crispy, about 5 to 7 minutes.

4. Remove the ground turkey from the skillet and place it in a bowl.

5. Add the remaining tablespoon of avocado oil to the pan, followed by the shallot, ginger, garlic, mushrooms, and water chestnuts. Cook, stirring, for 3 to 5 minutes, or until the mushrooms have cooked down to about a quarter in volume.

6. Add the ground turkey back into the pan, followed by the sauce. Stir so the sauce evenly coats the ground turkey and mushroom mixture. Mix in the cashews and ½ cup of the scallions.

7. Serve family-style with the ground turkey, lettuce leaves, pickled carrots, remaining scallions, and cilantro leaves in separate bowls.

8. To create a lettuce wrap, place 2 to 3 tablespoons of the turkey mixture inside a lettuce leaf and top with the pickled carrots and cilantro.

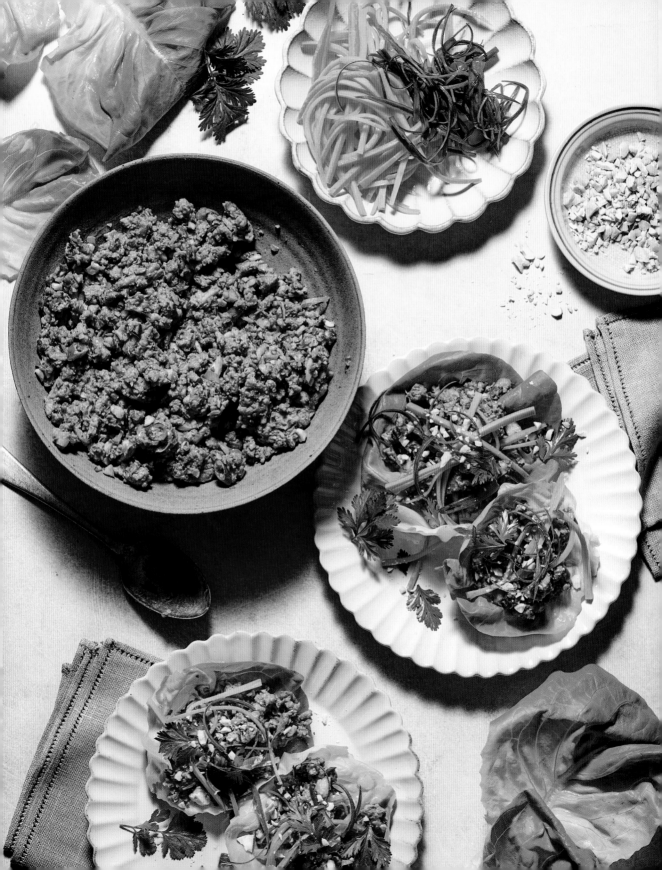

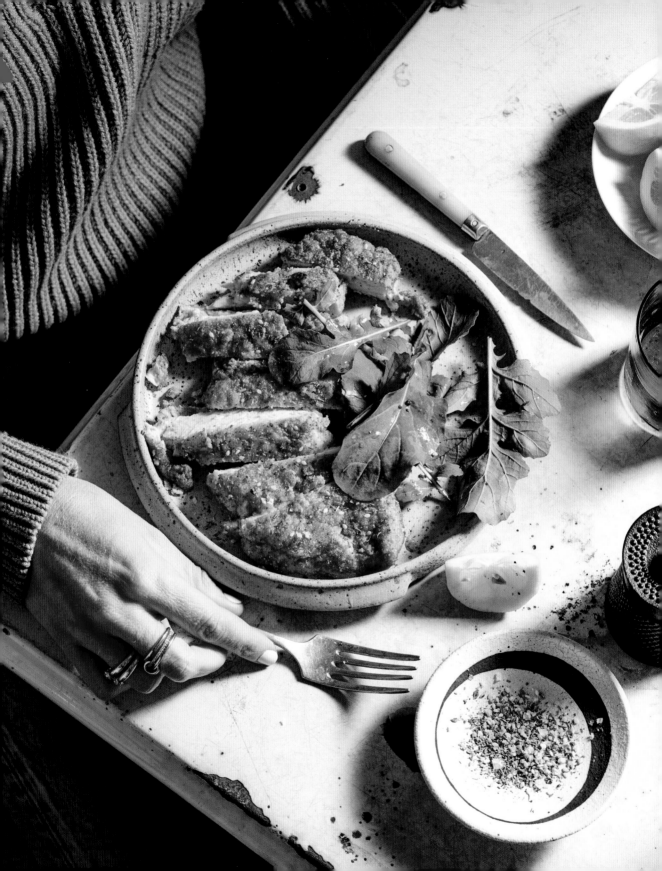

Zaatar-Crusted Chicken Cutlets with Arugula Salad

Brining the chicken first transforms this dish. While it's not 100 percent necessary, the brining process makes the chicken incredibly tender, juicy, and flavorful. Make sure to thoroughly dry the chicken before cooking so the crust stays intact.

SERVES 2 TO 4

FOR THE BRINE (OPTIONAL)
4 cups water

3 tablespoons sea salt

1 tablespoon black peppercorns

1 lemon, sliced

1 parsley sprig with leaves

FOR THE CHICKEN CUTLETS
1 pound boneless, skinless chicken breast

½ teaspoon salt

¼ teaspoon freshly ground black pepper

1 large egg

½ cup almond flour

2 tablespoons zaatar

1 teaspoon garlic powder

1 tablespoon avocado oil

FOR THE ARUGULA SALAD
4 cups arugula

2 tablespoons extra-virgin olive oil

½ teaspoon flaked sea salt, like Maldon

½ lemon

1. Make the brine. In a medium saucepan, add the water, salt, peppercorns, lemon slices, and parsley sprig, and bring to a boil, stirring to ensure all the salt is dissolved. Allow to cool completely, then submerge the chicken in the brine for at least 1 hour. Make sure the liquid is completely cooled at or below room temperature, or it could be a safety hazard.

2. Remove the chicken from the brine and place on a non-wooden surface. Dry the chicken completely with paper towels, then place each chicken breast into a separate Ziploc bag. Seal the bags and pound the chicken with a hammer or meat tenderizer until the chicken breasts are about ½-inch thick.

3. Remove the chicken from the Ziploc bags, season with salt and pepper, and set aside.

4. In a shallow bowl, whisk the egg. In a separate wide, shallow bowl, mix together the almond flour, zaatar, and garlic powder.

5. Dip the chicken breasts one by one in the egg, then in the flour mixture, and set aside.

6. In a large skillet, heat the avocado oil over medium-high heat. Add the chicken to the skillet and cook for 3 to 4 minutes on each side.

7. While the chicken is cooking, make the arugula salad. In a medium bowl, toss the arugula with the olive oil and sea salt.

8. Transfer the chicken to individual plates or a serving platter with a heaping portion of arugula, and squeeze the lemon over everything.

Chicken en Papillote

The term *en papillote* is French for "in a paper envelope," and describes this unique cooking technique where food is baked inside a pouch made of parchment paper, retaining the juices and flavors of the food during the cooking process. Cooking chicken by this method makes for a succulent and juicy dish that is just as good the next day as it is for dinner.

SERVES 2 TO 4

1 pound boneless, skinless chicken breasts

½ teaspoon sea salt

1 to 2 tablespoons extra-virgin olive oil

1 lemon, sliced into rounds

Fresh thyme (1 sprig thyme per chicken breast)

Note: To make this chicken extra juicy, use the brining technique from the Zaatar-Crusted Chicken Cutlets (page 155).

1. Preheat the oven to 350°F.

2. Make a parchment papillote for each chicken breast. Take a 12 x 12-inch sheet of parchment paper and fold it in half widthwise. Cut the parchment paper into the largest heart shape you can make. When you unfold the paper, it will be shaped like a heart with a fold in the middle.

3. Place the parchment paper flat on a cutting board, and put the chicken breast on one side of the fold. Season with a pinch of salt, brush with enough olive oil to lightly coat the chicken breast, about ½ tablespoon per chicken breast, and place a slice of lemon and a sprig of thyme on top.

4. Fold the other side of the parchment paper over the chicken breast and, starting with the point of the heart, fold little crimps to enclose the chicken in the parchment, leaving some room for the paper to expand while baking.

5. Repeat with the remaining chicken breasts.

6. Place the packets on a baking sheet and bake for 30 to 40 minutes, or until a thermometer inserted into the thickest part of the chicken reads 165°F.

Herbed Leg of Lamb

This recipe is great for a crowd alongside roasted vegetables, a simple salad, and whole grain. I love this dish for a holiday dinner or Sunday roast. It makes for equally satisfying leftovers!

SERVES 4 TO 6

1 (4- to 6-pound) bone-in leg of lamb (Ask your butcher to trim the fat for you.)

2 tablespoons fresh rosemary leaves

2 tablespoons fresh parsley leaves

8 to 10 olive oil–packed anchovies

4 garlic cloves, roughly chopped

1 tablespoon lemon zest

1 teaspoon freshly ground black pepper

¼ cup extra-virgin olive oil

1. Preheat the oven to 375°F.

2. Take the lamb out of the refrigerator at least 45 minutes before roasting to bring it to room temperature. Using a sharp knife, cut ten to twelve 1-inch-thick incisions throughout the lamb.

3. Using a blender, food processor, or mortar and pestle, make a paste of the rosemary, parsley, anchovies, garlic, lemon zest, black pepper, and olive oil.

4. Use your hands to massage the herb-anchovy mixture into the lamb, making sure to get it into the incisions.

5. Place the lamb in a roasting pan. Roast for 1 hour 45 minutes for medium. Use a meat thermometer to check doneness; medium should read 145° to 150°F.

Shepherd's Pie with Celery Root Top

My husband is British and loves a savory pie. I never quite understood it until I started experimenting with this dish. The celery root top is immensely flavorful and makes a great substitute for potatoes. If you can't find celery root, cauliflower will do the job!

SERVES 4 TO 6

2 pounds celery root, peeled and diced (about 6 cups)

1 pound ground lamb

1 teaspoon sea salt

½ teaspoon freshly ground black pepper

2 large carrots, peeled and diced

2 celery stalks, diced

½ medium onion, diced

2 garlic cloves, minced

1 tablespoon tomato paste

¼ cup peas, fresh or frozen

½ teaspoon paprika, plus more for garnish

½ teaspoon ground cumin

¼ teaspoon ground cinnamon

1 cup bone broth or stock

1 teaspoon gluten-free all-purpose flour

¼ cup full-fat unsweetened coconut milk

1. Preheat the oven to 350°F.

2. In a large stock pot, bring 2 quarts of generously salted water to a boil. Add the celery root, bring back to a boil, and then reduce the heat to medium. Cook the celery root until it is softened and a knife easily cuts through, about 7 to 10 minutes.

3. In a cast-iron skillet over medium heat, sauté the ground lamb, breaking it apart with a wooden spoon and stirring occasionally until fully cooked, about 6 to 8 minutes. Season with salt and pepper.

4. Remove the lamb from the skillet, and strain and discard excess fat, leaving just a thin coating that the vegetables will be cooked in.

5. To the same skillet over medium heat, add the carrots, celery, onion, and garlic, and sauté for 4 to 6 minutes.

6. Add the tomato paste and stir to combine. Add the peas, followed by the paprika, cumin, and cinnamon, and continue to cook. Season with salt and pepper.

7. Return the lamb to the skillet, stir to combine, then add the broth. Sprinkle the gluten-free flour on top and stir the mixture. Reduce the heat to low and allow the mixture to simmer.

8. Meanwhile, drain the celery root, then add the coconut milk and puree with a hand blender until smooth. Season with salt and pepper to taste.

9. Spread the celery root mash evenly over the lamb mixture in the skillet, and bake for 20 to 25 minutes, or until lightly browned on top and the gravy peeps through the sides.

10. Remove from the oven and sprinkle with paprika.

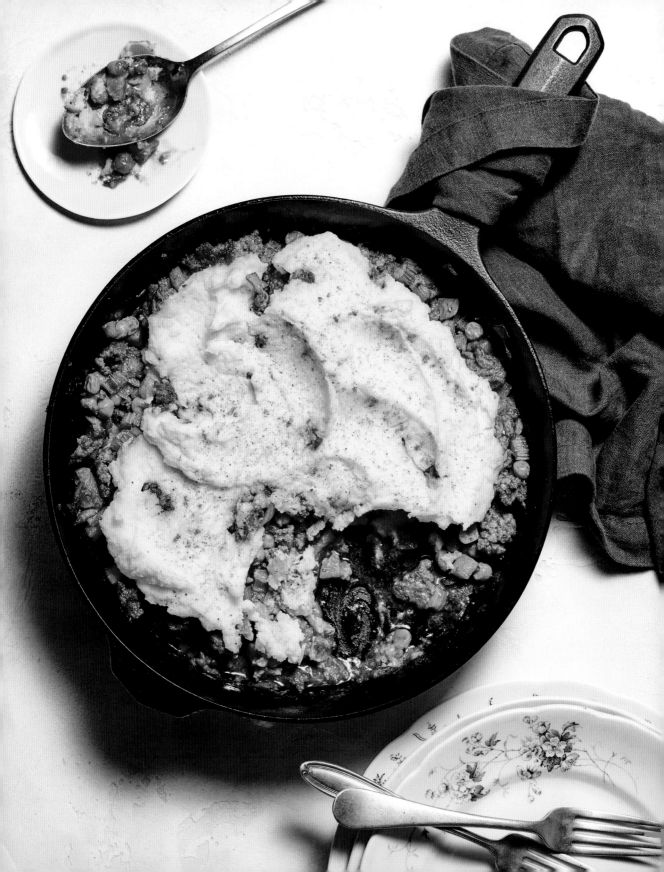

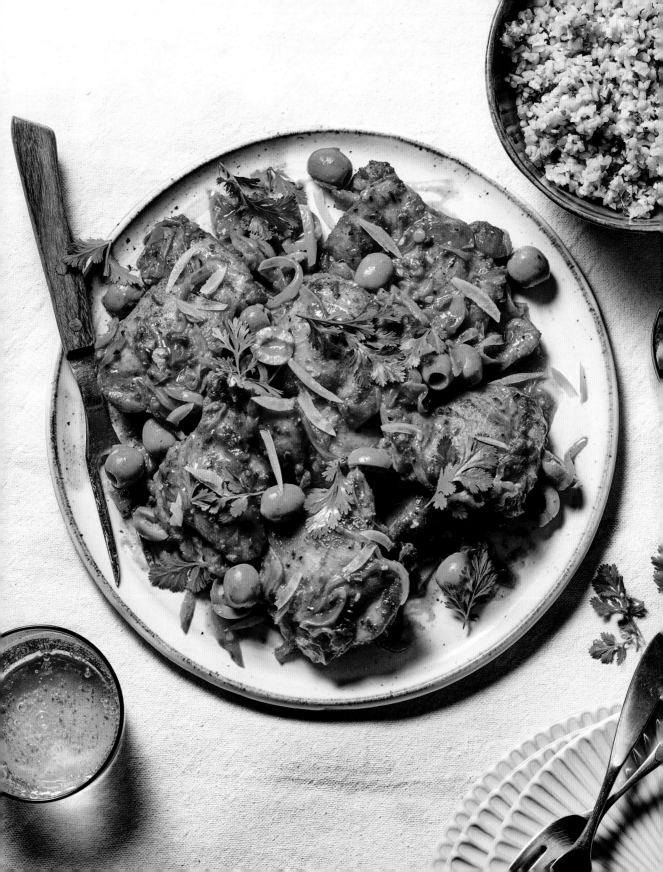

Spiced Chicken with Green Olives

This is my go-to dish to serve at a dinner party. It's easy to make ahead of time, is always a crowd-pleaser, and makes for great leftovers. I've literally never made it for friends and had them not ask for the recipe, so here you all go. Serve it with Spicy Roasted Broccoli Rabe (page 114) and Herbed Brown Rice & Cauliflower Pilaf (page 139).

SERVES 4 TO 6

1-inch piece ginger, peeled and diced

1 garlic clove, minced

2 tablespoons extra-virgin olive oil

Zest of 1 lemon

1 teaspoon sea salt

¼ teaspoon freshly ground black pepper

½ teaspoon ground turmeric

½ teaspoon ground cumin

½ teaspoon ground coriander

¼ teaspoon smoked paprika

1½ pounds boneless, skinless chicken thighs

1 large yellow onion, thinly sliced

1 cup chicken broth

1½ tablespoons lemon juice (from about ½ lemon)

1 teaspoon gluten-free all-purpose flour

½ cup pitted Castelvetrano olives, halved lengthwise

¼ cup chopped fresh cilantro (for garnish)

1. In a medium mixing bowl, add the ginger, garlic, olive oil, lemon zest, salt, pepper, turmeric, cumin, coriander, and paprika, and whisk to combine.

2. Add the chicken, stirring to coat thoroughly with spice mixture, and let it sit for 15 to 30 minutes.

3. Heat a large skillet over medium to high heat. Using tongs, add the chicken evenly across the bottom of the pan. Sear for 3 to 5 minutes on each side, or until lightly browned.

4. Remove the chicken from the pan and set aside. Reduce the heat to medium-low and add the onion. Cook, stirring occasionally, for 8 to 12 minutes, or until soft and lightly caramelized.

5. Pour the broth and juice into the pan, and sprinkle the flour on top. Stir everything to combine, bring to a simmer, and nestle the chicken back into the pan.

6. Let the mixture simmer uncovered for at least 10 minutes or up to an hour. The longer it simmers, the more tender the chicken will be.

7. Taste the broth and add salt and pepper as desired.

8. Scatter the olives evenly over the chicken and in the broth.

9. Garnish with the cilantro.

MEAT, POULTRY & SEAFOOD

Mediterranean Lamb Meatball Lettuce Wraps

Lamb has a slightly gamey taste, which is brightened up with fresh herbs, crunchy lettuce wraps, and a creamy lemon-tahini dressing. These meatballs also freeze well and are a great addition to pastas and bowls, so you may want to double your batch!

MAKES 12 TO 15 MEATBALLS

FOR THE MEATBALLS
1 cup spinach

1 medium shallot, peeled and roughly chopped

½ cup roughly chopped fresh parsley, leaves and stems

½ cup roughly chopped fresh basil, leaves and stems

2 garlic cloves, peeled and roughly chopped

Leaves from 3 thyme sprigs

1 pound ground lamb

1 teaspoon ground cumin

½ teaspoon sea salt

½ teaspoon freshly ground black pepper

FOR THE TAHINI DRESSING
2 tablespoons tahini

½ tablespoon water

2 tablespoons lemon juice

¼ cup extra-virgin olive oil

1 teaspoon sea salt

FOR ASSEMBLY
1 head butter lettuce, leaves separated and washed

1. Preheat the oven to 350°F and line a baking sheet with parchment paper.

2. In a food processor, pulse the spinach, shallot, parsley, basil, garlic, and thyme until finely chopped, scraping down the sides of the bowl with a spatula as needed.

3. In a medium bowl, combine the spinach mixture with the ground lamb. Season with the cumin, salt, and pepper, and mix with your hands until fully incorporated.

4. Heat a frying pan over medium heat.

5. Test your seasoning by pan-frying a mini meatball. Lamb is a fatty meat, so you do not need to oil the pan.

6. Use your hands to roll golf ball–size meatballs and add them to the frying pan one by one.

7. Use tongs to rotate the meatballs, browning on all sides, about 2 minutes per side, then place them on the prepared baking sheet. The meatballs should not be fully cooked, but browning them before baking will help lock in the moisture.

8. Bake the meatballs for 15 minutes.

9. While the meatballs are baking, make the tahini dressing. In a bowl, combine the tahini and the water, and whisk to loosen. Add the lemon juice, whisk to combine, then slowly add in the olive oil, whisking until smooth. Season with salt to taste.

10. When ready to serve, lay one meatball on top of a lettuce leaf, and drizzle with the tahini dressing. Repeat with the rest of the meatballs.

Grilled Skirt Steak Piled with Shiitake Mushrooms & Onions

All-grass-fed is the healthiest option when buying beef; it has more protein, antioxidants, and B vitamins than commercial beef and an ideal ratio of omega-3 to omega-6 fatty acids. With this level of nutrient density, you don't need as much to feel satisfied; three to four ounces should suffice!

SERVES 4

1 garlic clove, minced

1 teaspoon lime zest

2 tablespoons lime juice, plus more for garnish

1 tablespoon tamari

2 tablespoons extra-virgin olive oil, divided, plus more as needed

1 pound grass-fed skirt steak

1 medium yellow onion, thinly sliced

Sea salt and freshly ground black pepper, to taste

3 to 4 cups shiitake mushrooms, sliced

Chopped parsley leaves (for garnish)

1. In a medium bowl, mix together the garlic, lime zest, lime juice, tamari, and 1 tablespoon of the olive oil. Add the steak and allow it to marinate for at least 30 minutes but up to 5 hours.

2. In a large skillet over medium heat, heat 1 tablespoon of the olive oil. Add the onion, season with salt and pepper, and sauté for 3 to 5 minutes, or until softened.

3. Add the mushrooms plus a pinch more salt, and continue to sauté for another 5 to 10 minutes, stirring occasionally.

4. Heat a grill or grill plan to high, then cook the marinated steak on the grill for 3 to 4 minutes on each side for medium, and allow it to rest for 5 to 10 minutes.

5. Slice the skirt steak and arrange it on a platter topped with the onions and mushrooms. Garnish with a squeeze of lime juice and some parsley.

Spaghetti with Caramelized Onions Collard Greens, & Bacon

This is a crowd-pleaser for all the bacon lovers out there. In this recipe, onions and collard greens are thinly sliced to resemble noodles and cooked in bacon fat. Yes, you read that right: bacon fat. When buying bacon, make sure to get organic, uncured bacon without any added sugars or nitrates.

SERVES 4

1 (1-pound) package organic, uncured, sugar-free bacon

1 medium yellow onion, halved and thinly sliced

4 ounces gluten-free spaghetti

2 bundles collard greens or Swiss chard, stems removed and sliced into ½-inch ribbons (about 4 cups)

2 garlic cloves, minced

Zest of 1 lemon

Juice of 1 lemon, divided

Sea salt and freshly ground black pepper, to taste

1 tablespoon extra-virgin olive oil

Grated Pecorino cheese (optional)

1. Heat a large skillet to medium-high, and line two dinner plates with paper towels. Chop the bacon into bite-size pieces and cook in the skillet until crispy, stirring frequently about 5 to 7 minutes.

2. Transfer the bacon to paper towel–lined plates and discard all but 2 tablespoons of the bacon fat.

3. In the same skillet over medium-low heat, heat the reserved bacon fat. Add the onion and cook until caramelized, 12 to 15 minutes, stirring frequently.

4. While the onions are caramelizing, cook the pasta according to package instructions.

5. To the skillet, add the collard greens, garlic, lemon zest, half of the lemon juice, salt, and pepper, and sauté until the collard greens have wilted, about 5 minutes.

6. Return the bacon to the pan, followed by the cooked pasta. The ratio of pasta to onions and collard greens should be 1:2.

7. Season with salt and pepper to taste, drizzle with olive oil, and add more lemon juice as desired. Serve with shredded Pecorino, if using.

Harissa Salmon

Originally from Tunisia, harissa is a chili paste or sauce that adds a wildly smoky, spicy flavor and brings this simple roasted salmon to a new dimension.

SERVES 3 TO 4

1 pound wild salmon fillet

2 tablespoons extra-virgin olive oil

1 teaspoon harissa paste

1 tablespoon fresh lemon juice

½ teaspoon sea salt

Fresh dill and mint (for garnish)

1. Preheat the oven to 325°F. Remove the salmon from the refrigerator to bring it to room temperature.

2. In a small saucepan or butter warmer, heat the olive oil, harissa paste, and lemon juice, and whisk until combined.

3. Place the salmon on a baking dish and season with salt.

4. Pour the harissa–olive oil mixture over the salmon, and bake for 15 to 20 minutes.

5. Serve garnished with fresh dill and mint.

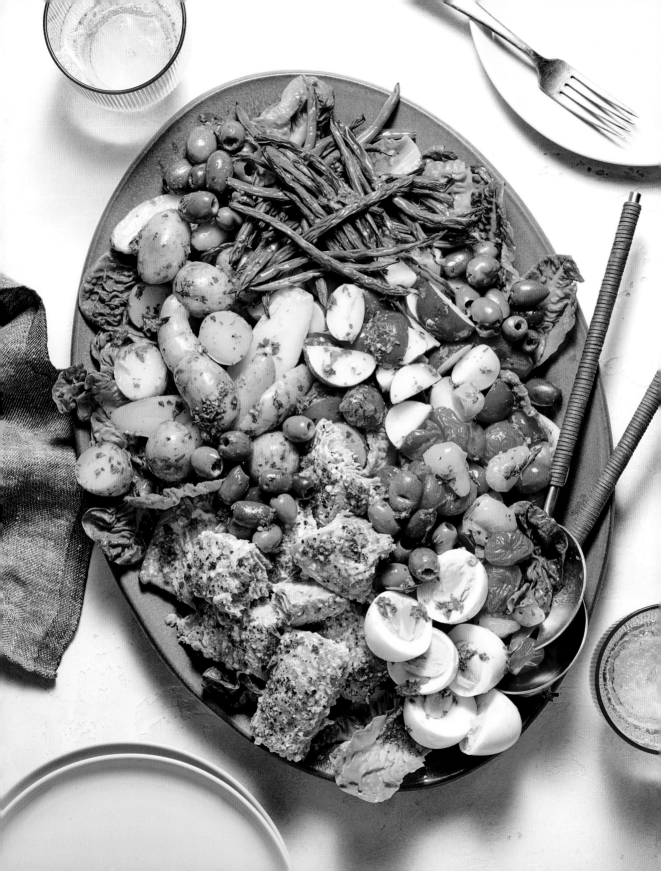

Salmon Niçoise

When entertaining, I always look to make a dish that allows me to spend time with my guests, not in the kitchen. This dish requires a little bit of upfront prep, but the finished product is more of an assembly job, which makes it perfect for a brunch or dinner party. But rest assured, when you present this family-style dish, everyone will get their cameras out.

SERVES 4 TO 6

1 pound fingerling potatoes

Sea salt, to taste

1 pound cherry tomatoes

½ pound haricot verts, trimmed

¼ cup plus 3 to 4 tablespoons extra-virgin olive oil

Freshly ground black pepper, to taste

3 large eggs

1 cup fresh parsley, leaves and stems

4 to 6 fresh basil leaves

½ garlic clove

6 oil-packed anchovies

1 teaspoon Dijon mustard

1 tablespoon lemon juice

1½ to 2 pounds salmon fillets

2 heads little gem lettuce, leaves washed and separated

1 bunch radishes, quartered

½ cup mixed Greek olives

Pinch of Maldon sea salt

Note: You can prep the salad up to 1 day in advance and store it in the refrigerator until ready to serve.

1. In a large pot, add the potatoes, cover with water, and season with a generous amount of sea salt. Bring to a boil over a high heat and cook for about 5 minutes, or until a knife easily cuts through the potato.

2. While the potatoes are cooking, create an ice bath in a medium-size mixing bowl. Drain the potatoes, and place them in the ice bath to stop the cooking process. Once cool, halve the fingerling potatoes and set aside.

3. Preheat the oven to 350°F. Place the cherry tomatoes and haricot verts on a baking sheet. Cover with 1 to 2 tablespoons of the olive oil and a generous pinch of sea salt and black pepper. Roast for 20 to 25 minutes, or until the tomatoes burst and are lightly browned. Set aside to cool.

4. In a medium saucepan, add the eggs and cover with water. Bring to a boil, then turn off the heat and allow the eggs to cook for 7 minutes, then place in an ice bath.

5. Make the dressing. In a food processor, add the parsley, basil, garlic, anchovies, Dijon mustard, lemon juice, and ¼ cup of the olive oil, and pulse until combined, but not pureed. Set the dressing aside.

6. Heat the grill or preheat the oven to 350°F. Season both sides of the salmon fillet with kosher salt and black pepper, and rub with a tablespoon of the olive oil. Grill or bake the salmon for 15 to 25 minutes, or until cooked through.

7. While the salmon is cooking, assemble the salad. Dress the little gem leaves, radishes, and fingerling potatoes individually with a little olive oil and kosher salt. Then, on a large platter, arrange the little gem leaves, radishes, Greek olives, tomatoes, haricot verts, and fingerling potatoes.

8. Peel and halve the eggs and add to the platter, leaving room for the salmon.

9. When the salmon is done, add it to the platter, drizzle the herbed dressing all over, and season with the Maldon sea salt. Serve family-style warm or cool.

Spiced Tomato & Shrimp Bisque

A warming tomato and coconut bisque (a variation of which also features in the soup section) is used as a poaching liquid to make succulent shrimp. Paired with baby kale leaves and grounding brown rice, it creates a satisfying, hearty, and nutrient-rich dish that hits the spot.

SERVES 4

2 tablespoons avocado oil

1 medium shallot, roughly chopped

2 garlic cloves, peeled and roughly chopped

1 thumb-size piece ginger, roughly chopped

1 medium carrot, roughly chopped

¼ fresh cayenne pepper, deseeded and roughly chopped, or ¼ teaspoon ground cayenne pepper (optional)

1 (15-ounce) can diced tomatoes

1 (13.5-ounce) can full-fat, unsweetened coconut milk

1 (16-ounce) jar roasted red peppers

½ teaspoon ground cumin

½ teaspoon ground coriander

¼ teaspoon ground turmeric

Juice of 1 lime, plus lime wedges for serving

Salt and freshly ground black pepper, to taste

2 handfuls baby kale or roughly chopped dinosaur kale

1 pound jumbo wild shrimp, peeled and deveined

1 to 2 cups cooked brown rice (for serving)

1 handful fresh cilantro (for serving)

1 handful fresh basil (for serving)

1. In a large stock pot or Dutch oven, heat the avocado oil over medium-high heat.

2. Add the shallot, garlic, ginger, carrot, and cayenne pepper to the pot. Cook, stirring, for 3 to 5 minutes.

3. Add the tomatoes and their juices, coconut milk, and roasted red peppers to the pot. Reduce the heat and bring to a simmer. Add the cumin, coriander, turmeric, and the juice of 1 lime. Let the mixture simmer for 10 to 30 minutes.

4. Remove the bisque from the heat and using a hand blender, puree until smooth (if you don't have a hand blender, you can transfer the contents to a standing blender). Season with salt and pepper to taste.

5. Return the bisque to the pot and bring to a simmer. Add the kale and cook until wilted, about 5 minutes.

6. When ready to serve, add the shrimp and cook, stirring frequently, for 4 to 5 minutes, or until the shrimp are pink and cooked through.

7. Serve with the rice, cilantro, basil, and a wedge of lime.

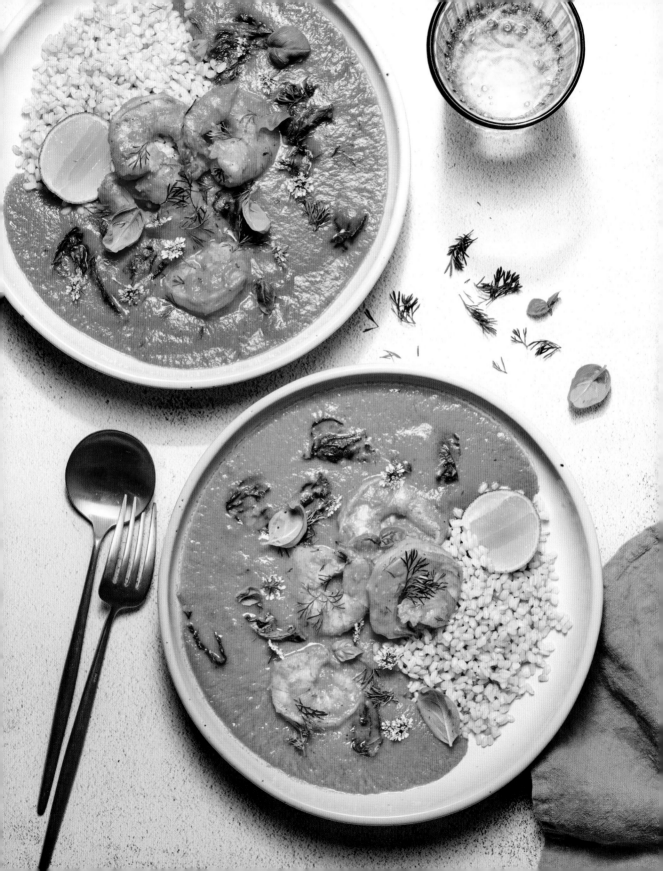

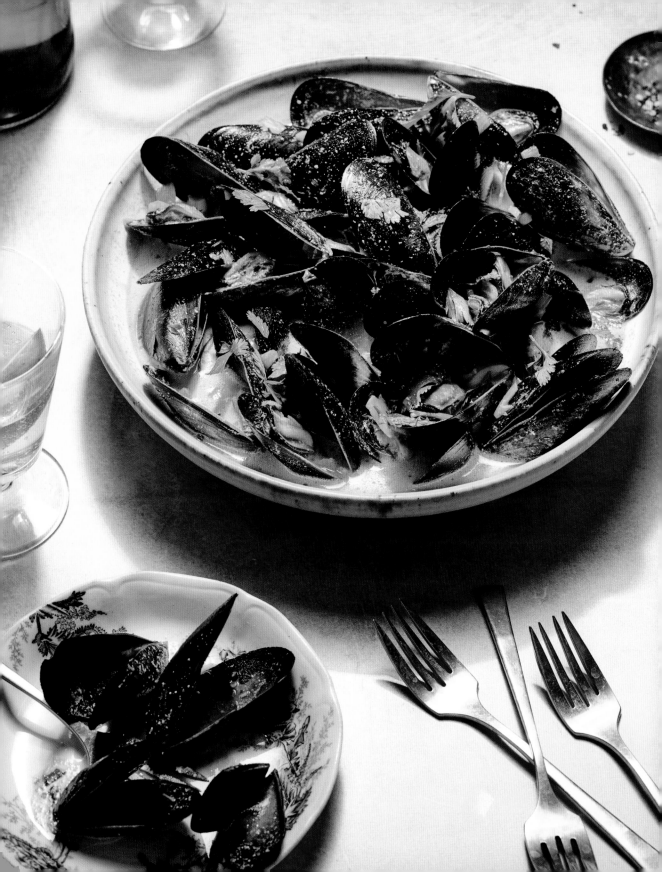

Coconut-Saffron Mussels

Saffron is the world's most luxurious spice. Known for its uplifting properties, saffron has been dubbed "nature's Prozac" and has been used to treat depression, anxiety, insomnia, and more. It is outrageously expensive (around $5,000 a pound!), but luckily a very little bit goes a long way. In this recipe, just a few threads of this exquisite spice infuse the coconut broth with immense flavor.

SERVES 2 TO 4

1½ pounds mussels

2 tablespoons extra-virgin
    olive oil

1 medium shallot, diced

1 garlic clove, minced

Pinch of saffron

¼ teaspoon ground turmeric

½ teaspoon red pepper flakes
    (optional)

Sea salt and freshly ground
    black pepper, to taste

1 (13.5-ounce) can full-fat
    unsweetened coconut milk

¾ cup clam juice

¼ cup chopped fresh cilantro
    (for garnish)

1. Wash the mussels in cool water and debeard. Discard any mussels that are cracked or have already opened.

2. In a Dutch oven, heat the olive oil over medium heat.

3. Add the shallot and garlic, and sauté for a few minutes.

4. Add the saffron, turmeric, red pepper flakes (if using), and a pinch of salt and pepper. Stir to combine, and cook until the mixture is fragrant, about 3 to 4 minutes.

5. Add the coconut milk and clam juice, and bring to a simmer.

6. Add the mussels, and cook, covered. Shake the pan and stir the mussels every minute or so until all the shells have opened, about 5 to 7 minutes.

7. Serve immediately garnished with the cilantro.

Cod Puttanesca

Puttanesca is an Italian sauce that was invented sometime around World War II and consists of olives, capers, garlic, chili pepper, anchovies, tomatoes, and olive oil. Originally it was meant for pasta, but its rich and dynamic flavor profile perfectly complements this flaky white fish.

SERVES 2 TO 4

2 tablespoons extra-virgin olive oil

½ medium white onion, quartered and sliced

1 fennel bulb, quartered and sliced

2 garlic cloves

5 oil-packed anchovies, drained

1 (28-ounce) can diced tomatoes

½ tablespoon red pepper flakes

½ cup olive oil–cured black olives, halved

2 tablespoons capers, drained

Leaves from 2 thyme sprigs

Sea salt and freshly ground black pepper, to taste

1½ pounds cod, cut into approximately 4-ounce pieces

1. In a cast-iron skillet, heat the olive oil over medium heat.

2. Add the onion, fennel, garlic, and anchovies, and cook, stirring frequently, for 3 to 5 minutes.

3. Add the tomatoes, red pepper flakes, olives, capers, and thyme leaves, and bring the mixture to a simmer. Season with salt and pepper to taste.

4. Nestle the cod into the sauce and cover with a lid or aluminum foil. Cook for 10 to 15 minutes, or until the fish is opaque and cooked through.

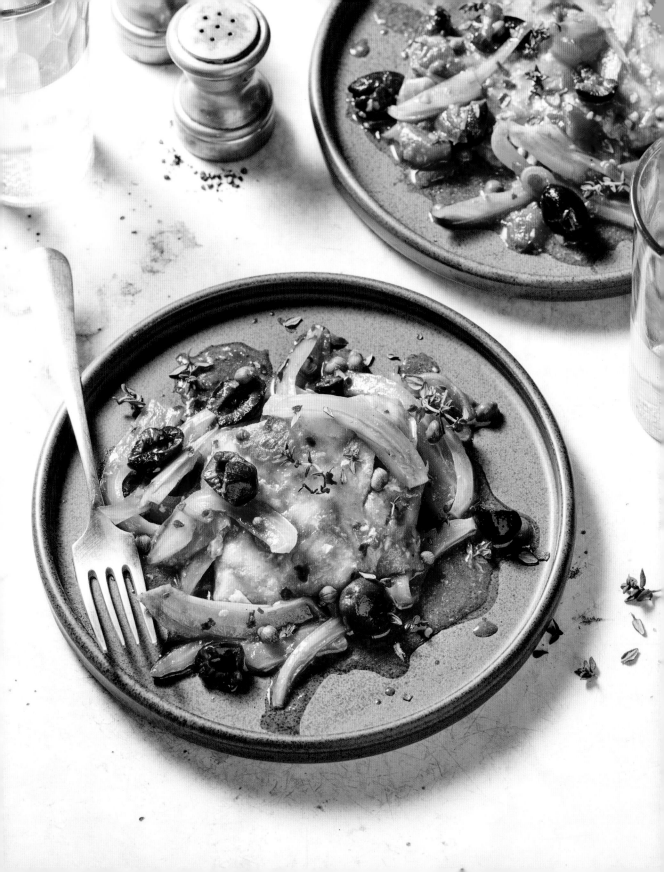

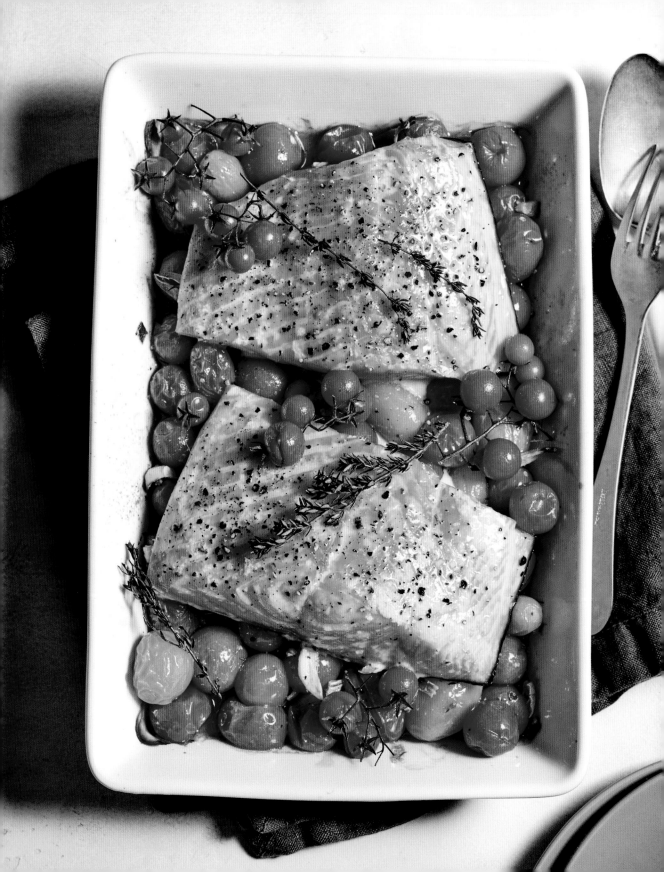

Roasted Salmon with Cherry Tomatoes & Shallots

A simple way to elevate salmon that is suitable for meal prep, weeknight dinner, or a Saturday-night soiree.

SERVES 3 TO 4

2 cups cherry tomatoes

1 medium shallot, diced

1 garlic clove, sliced

2 tablespoons extra-virgin olive oil

2 thyme sprigs

Sea salt and freshly ground black pepper, to taste

1 to 1½ pounds salmon, either a steak or sliced in 3- to 4-ounce portions

1. Preheat the oven to 350°F.

2. On a large baking sheet, place the cherry tomatoes, shallot, and garlic.

3. Cover the tomatoes in the olive oil, add the thyme, and season generously with salt and pepper.

4. Bake for 30 minutes, or until the tomatoes pop. If they haven't popped after 30 minutes, pierce the un-popped tomatoes with a fork.

5. Season the salmon with salt and pepper, then nestle the salmon on the baking sheet in between the tomatoes.

6. Return the baking sheet to the oven and bake for an additional 12 to 20 minutes, or until the salmon is flaky.

Soup

The Original Green Soup

This is original Reset recipe boasts more than six different types of plants, anti-inflammatory spices, and a soothing broth base. Top with Seeded Crackers (page 193) for extra crunch.

SERVES 4

2 tablespoons extra-virgin olive oil, plus more for garnish

1 medium yellow onion, roughly chopped

1 thumb-size piece ginger, roughly chopped

2 garlic cloves, roughly chopped

4 cups leafy greens (Try to include at least two different types, such as kale, beet greens, arugula, Swiss chard, spinach, watercress, etc.)

1 bunch fresh parsley, stems included, roughly chopped

1 teaspoon ground turmeric

4 cups chicken bone broth or vegetable broth

Water, to cover (about 2 cups)

Sea salt and freshly ground black pepper, to taste

1 tablespoon lemon juice

1 tablespoon sesame seeds (for serving)

Pinch of Maldon sea salt (for serving)

1. In a Dutch oven, heat the extra-virgin olive oil over medium heat. Add the onion, ginger, and garlic, and cook, stirring until fragrant about 1 minute.

2. Add the leafy greens, parsley, and turmeric and stir for a minute longer.

3. Add the broth and enough water to cover the vegetables. Let it simmer for 20 to 30 minutes (do not bring to a boil, as it will destroy some of the nutrients from the greens). Use a handheld blender or transfer the mixture to a high-speed blender and puree until smooth.

4. Season as desired with salt and pepper, and serve with a squeeze of lemon juice, the sesame seeds, a splash of the olive oil, and Maldon sea salt.

White Bean & Leek Soup

Using dried cannellini beans is integral to the recipe. It won't be the same with canned beans. Make sure to soak them overnight to get the best texture and flavor.

SERVES 4

2 tablespoons extra-virgin olive oil

1 leek, washed and roughly chopped (white parts only)

2 celery stalks, roughly chopped

2 garlic cloves, peeled and roughly chopped

1 cup dry cannellini beans, soaked overnight

4 cups chicken or vegetable broth

1 sprig fresh rosemary

2 sprigs fresh thyme

Sea salt and freshly ground black pepper, to taste

Pistachio Pistou (page 220) (for garnish)

1. Heat a stock pot or Dutch oven over medium. Add the olive oil, leek, celery, and garlic. Cook, stirring occasionally, until fragrant and slightly translucent, 4 to 5 minutes.

2. Drain the beans and add them to the pot, along with the broth. Bring to a simmer, then add the rosemary and thyme.

3. Allow to cook for 60 to 90 minutes, or until the beans are soft and mushy.

4. Remove the thyme and rosemary sprigs and use a handheld blender or transfer the mixture to a high-speed blender. Puree until smooth.

5. Season with salt and pepper, and garnish with Pistachio Pistou, as desired.

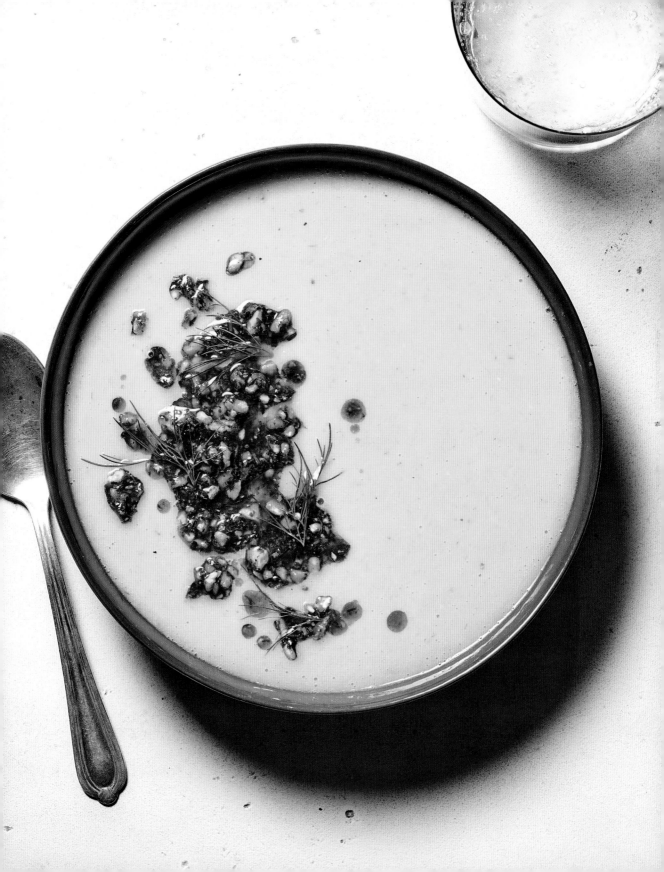

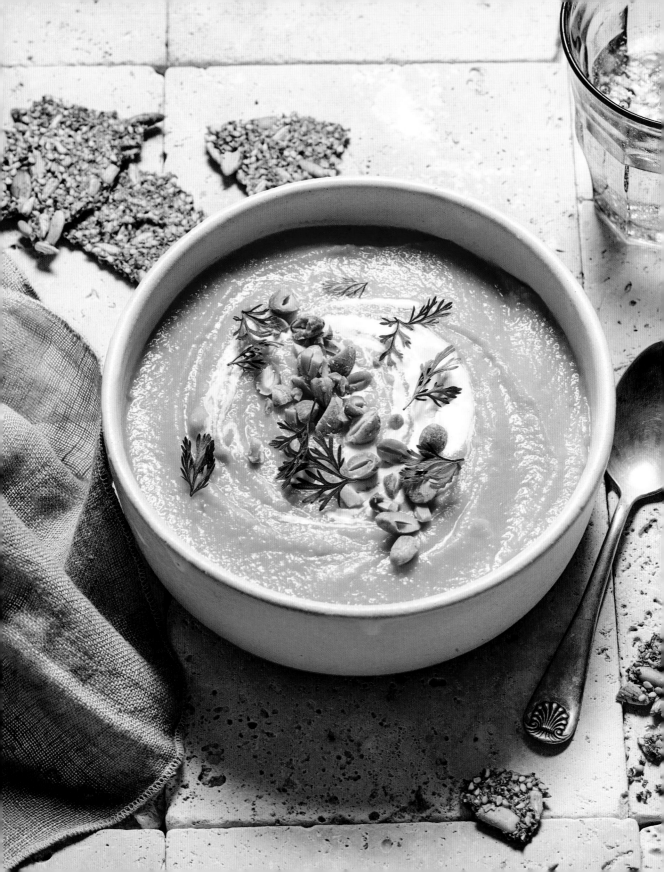

Jazzy Carrot & Parsnip Soup

The garnish on this soup gets a crunch from sacha inchi seeds, a Peruvian seed that is rich in protein, essential fatty acids, vitamin E, vitamin A, omega-3, and fiber. They also make a great snack, so if you've never heard of sacha inchi seeds before, they're worth a try! While you might not be able to find them at your local grocery store, they're readily available at online grocers and specialty foods shops.

SERVES 4

2 tablespoons extra-virgin olive oil, plus more for garnish

1 medium yellow onion, roughly chopped

1-inch piece fresh ginger, roughly chopped

2 garlic cloves, roughly chopped

1 teaspoon ground cumin

1 teaspoon ground turmeric

6 medium carrots, peeled and cut into 1-inch pieces, tops reserved for garnish

3 medium-size parsnips, peeled and cut into 1-inch pieces

5 cups bone broth

1 cup coconut milk, plus more for garnish

Sea salt, to taste

Sacha inchi seeds or toasted almonds (for garnish)

1. In a medium or large Dutch oven, heat the olive oil over medium heat.

2. Add the onion, ginger, and garlic, and sauté until fragrant, about 3 minutes.

3. Add the cumin and turmeric, then the carrots and parsnips, and cook, stirring, for a few minutes more.

4. Pour in the bone broth and coconut milk, and bring to a simmer. Cook, covered, at a simmer for about 20 minutes, or until carrots and parsnips are extremely tender.

5. Use a hand blender or transfer the contents to a high-speed blender and blend until smooth.

6. Season with salt as desired. Serve with a drizzle of the coconut milk and olive oil. Garnish with carrot top greens and sacha inchi seeds or toasted almonds.

Spiced Tomato & Coconut Bisque

This soup is like tomato bisque on a tropical vacation. Vibrant spices, ginger, garlic, and a little heat from a fresh cayenne pepper brighten up this rendition of a classic soup and add dimension, flavor, and (of course) nutrition. If you can't find fresh cayenne pepper, a dash of ground cayenne will do the trick. Feel free to adjust the seasoning according to your preference.

SERVES 4

2 tablespoons avocado oil

1 medium shallot, roughly chopped

2 garlic cloves, peeled and roughly chopped

1 thumb-size piece ginger, peeled and roughly chopped

1 medium carrot, peeled and roughly chopped

¼ fresh cayenne pepper, deseeded and roughly chopped (optional)

1 (14.5-ounce) can diced tomatoes with their juices

1 (13.5-ounce) can full-fat unsweetened coconut milk

1 (16-ounce) jar roasted red peppers

2 cups chicken or vegetable broth

½ teaspoon ground cumin

½ teaspoon ground coriander

¼ teaspoon ground turmeric

2 limes

Sea salt and freshly ground black pepper, to taste

Fresh basil and cilantro (for garnish)

1. In a large stock pot or Dutch oven, heat the avocado oil over medium-high heat.

2. Add the shallot, garlic, ginger, carrot, and cayenne pepper to the pot. Cook, stirring, for 3 to 5 minutes.

3. Add the tomatoes, coconut milk, peppers, and broth to the pot, and bring to a simmer. Add the cumin, coriander, turmeric, and the juice of 1 lime. Let simmer for 10 to 30 minutes.

4. Turn the heat off and, using a hand blender, puree until smooth (if you don't have a hand blender, you can transfer the contents to a standing blender). Season with salt and pepper as desired.

5. Serve hot with a squeeze of lime juice from the remaining lime, and garnished with the basil and cilantro.

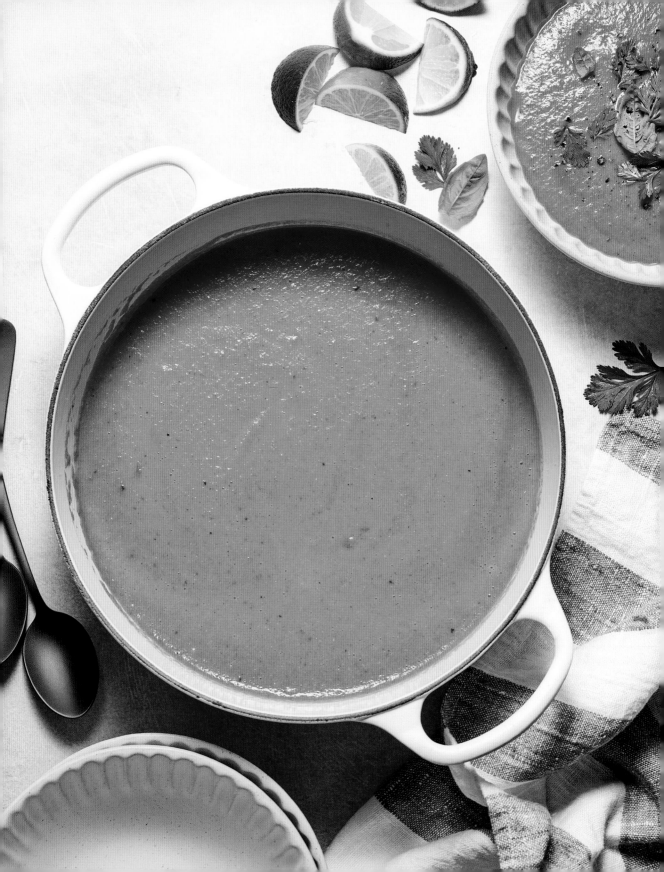

Harissa-Spiced Acorn Squash Soup

Acorn squash is one of my favorite winter squashes, not only for its sweet and buttery taste, but also because you can eat the skin, which makes cooking this soup a breeze (and with minimal waste!).

SERVES 4

2 medium acorn squash

¼ cup plus 1 tablespoon
coconut oil

Sea salt and freshly ground
black pepper, to taste

1 medium yellow onion,
roughly chopped

2 garlic cloves, peeled and
roughly chopped

2 tablespoons harissa paste

4 cups bone or vegetable
broth

Rosemary, fresh or dried
(for garnish)

1. Preheat the oven to 350°F.

2. Cut the acorn squash into 1-inch squares and scoop out the seeds. Place the squash on a parchment paper–lined baking sheet.

3. Melt ¼ cup of the coconut oil and pour it evenly over the squash. Season with salt and pepper, and roast for 40 minutes, or until tender.

4. In a Dutch oven, heat the remaining tablespoon of coconut oil over medium heat.

5. Add the onion and garlic, and cook, stirring, for 2 to 3 minutes.

6. Add the roasted squash and harissa paste to the onion mixture, and continue to cook, stirring, for 1 to 2 minutes more. Pour in the broth. Bring the mixture to a simmer and allow to cook for 15 to 20 minutes.

7. Use a handheld blender or transfer contents to a high-speed blender and puree until smooth. Season with salt and pepper. Serve garnished with rosemary.

Coconut-Curry & Lime Soup

Zucchini is very creamy when cooked and pureed, which gives this soup a luscious texture that pairs great with coconut milk and ground curry.

SERVES 4

1 tablespoon avocado oil

1 medium yellow onion, roughly chopped

1 garlic clove

1 medium zucchini, roughly chopped

1 bunch rainbow chard, roughly chopped

1 tablespoon curry powder

4 cups bone broth

2 cups coconut milk

Juice of 1 lime

Sea salt and freshly ground black pepper, to taste

¼ cup toasted coconut flakes (for garnish)

¼ cup pumpkin seeds, toasted (for garnish)

1. In a medium to large saucepan or Dutch oven, heat the avocado oil over medium heat. Add the onion and garlic, and cook, stirring, until fragrant, about 3 minutes.

2. Add the zucchini and rainbow chard, and sauté for 3 to 5 minutes. Add the curry powder, and stir to combine.

3. Pour the bone broth and coconut milk over the vegetables and bring to a simmer. Cover with a lid, reduce the heat to low, and allow the soup to continue simmering for 20 to 30 minutes.

4. Add in the lime juice, and blend the mixture with a handheld blender or transfer the contents to a high-speed blender to puree.

5. Season with salt and pepper to taste, and serve garnished with the toasted coconut flakes and pumpkin seeds.

Roasted Cauliflower & Garlic Soup

The secret ingredient in this soup is miso paste, which not only provides probiotic value, but also has a rich, salty, umami flavor. Probiotics are live cultures, and will die at a high heat, so make sure to only simmer, and not boil, your soup.

SERVES 4

1 head cauliflower, including leaves and stems, roughly chopped

1 medium yellow onion, roughly chopped

2 garlic cloves, roughly chopped

5 sprigs fresh thyme

2 tablespoons extra-virgin olive oil, plus more for garnish

Sea salt and freshly ground black pepper, to taste

4 cups bone broth

2 cups filtered water

1 tablespoon miso paste

Maldon sea salt (for garnish)

1. Preheat the oven to 350°F and line a baking sheet with parchment paper.

2. On the prepared baking sheet, spread the cauliflower, onion, garlic, and thyme in an even layer, and lightly coat with the olive oil, salt, and pepper. Roast for 45 minutes, or until browned.

3. Add the roasted vegetables to a blender with the broth, water, and miso paste, and blend until smooth.

4. Transfer the soup to a large pot and warm over low heat. Season with more salt and pepper as desired and top with a drizzle of olive oil and Maldon sea salt.

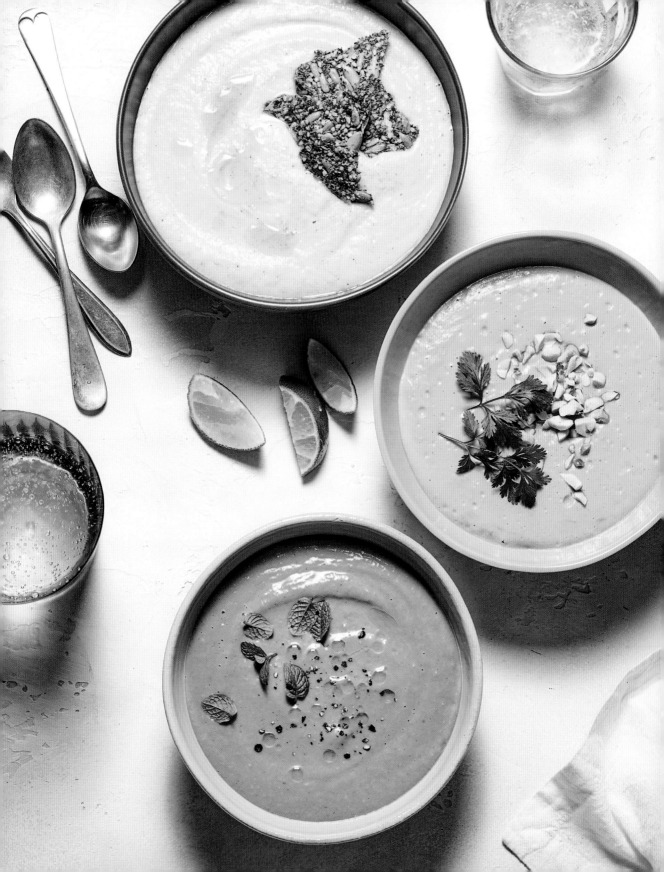

West African Peanut Soup

The flavors in this hearty and warming soup are explosive! To make into a larger meal, add shredded chicken and baby kale to the soup, and serve with brown rice.

SERVES 4

2 tablespoons avocado oil

1 medium yellow onion, roughly chopped

2 garlic cloves, peeled and roughly chopped

1-inch piece ginger, peeled and roughly chopped

1 medium carrot, peeled and roughly chopped

1 medium sweet potato, peeled and roughly chopped

1 tablespoon red curry paste

1 tablespoon tomato paste

½ cup creamy peanut butter

4 cups chicken bone broth

Sea salt and freshly ground black pepper, to taste

Juice of 1 lime

¼ cup chopped peanuts (for garnish)

¼ cup chopped fresh cilantro (for garnish)

1. In a Dutch oven, heat the avocado oil over medium heat.

2. Add the onion, garlic, ginger, carrot, and sweet potato, and sauté until fragrant, about 3 minutes.

3. Stir in the red curry paste and tomato paste, then add the peanut butter.

4. Pour the broth over the vegetable mixture and bring to a simmer. Allow the vegetables to gently cook in the broth until they are soft, about 25 minutes.

5. Transfer the contents to a high-speed blender or use a hand blender to blend until smooth. Season with salt and pepper to taste, and thin with water, ¼ cup at a time, until the soup is at your desired consistency and flavor.

6. Add the lime juice and serve garnished with chopped peanuts and cilantro.

Fresh Pea & Mint Soup

I enjoy this soup cold as much as I do hot, which means it's great for leftovers. Good-quality olive oil and sea salt accentuate the flavor of the peas and mint.

SERVES 4

4 cups peas, fresh and blanched or frozen and thawed

2 garlic cloves

2 cups spinach

1 ripe avocado, peeled and pit removed

3 cups unsweetened almond milk

3 cups filtered water

15 to 20 fresh mint leaves

2 tablespoons extra-virgin olive oil, plus more for garnish

Sea salt and freshly ground black pepper, to taste

Maldon sea salt (for garnish)

1. In a high-speed blender, combine the peas, garlic, spinach, avocado, almond milk, water, mint, and olive oil, and blend until smooth.

2. Season generously with salt and pepper to taste.

3. Serve chilled, at room temperature, or heated, with a drizzle of olive oil and a sprinkle of Maldon sea salt.

Broccoli Soup with "Cheesy" Cashew Cream

A creamy cashew blend takes this simple soup to a new level with the addition of nutritional yeast: a plant-based powerhouse rich in vitamin B12 and protein that has a naturally cheesy flavor.

SERVES 4

2 tablespoons extra-virgin olive oil

1 cup chopped leeks, whites only (from 1 medium leek)

2 cups broccoli (stems and florets), roughly chopped

2 garlic cloves

4 cups bone, chicken, or vegetable broth

Sea salt and freshly ground black pepper, to taste

1 cup raw, unsalted cashews, soaked in filtered water overnight or in hot water for 30 minutes

½ cup filtered water

Juice of 1 lemon

1 teaspoon nutritional yeast

1. In a Dutch oven, heat the olive oil over medium heat.

2. Add the leeks, broccoli, and garlic, and sauté for 3 minutes.

3. Pour the broth over the vegetables and bring to a simmer. Allow to cook over low heat until the broccoli is soft, about 30 minutes.

4. Use a handheld blender or transfer the contents to a high-speed blender and puree until smooth. Season with salt and pepper as desired.

5. To make the cashew cream, drain the cashews and add them to a high-speed blender with the water, lemon juice, nutritional yeast, and a generous pinch of salt. Blend until smooth.

6. Serve the soup with a tablespoon of cashew cream drizzled on top.

Snacks, Sweets & Baked Goods

Nut & Seed Protein Bread

This is a multifaceted loaf. It's a great complement to a meal, alongside eggs or a salad, or it can be a vehicle for toppings, like avocado, nut butter, or Chocolate Hazelnut Spread (page 212). Because of the high protein content of the nuts and seeds, it is a great snack for The Reset and beyond.

MAKES 1 LOAF

2 cups almond flour

½ cup coconut flour

½ cup ground flaxseeds

⅓ cup hemp seeds

⅓ cup pumpkin seeds

⅓ cup sunflower seeds

⅓ cup chopped walnuts

1 teaspoon baking soda

1 teaspoon sea salt

6 large eggs

½ cup extra-virgin olive oil, plus more for greasing the loaf pan

2 tablespoons apple cider vinegar

½ medium zucchini, grated

1. Preheat the oven to 350°F, line a 9-inch loaf pan with parchment paper, and grease the sides with olive oil.

2. In a large mixing bowl, add the almond flour, coconut flour, flaxseeds, hemp seeds, pumpkin seeds, sunflower seeds, walnuts, baking soda, and sea salt. Mix to combine and set aside.

3. In a separate bowl, whisk together the eggs, olive oil, apple cider vinegar, and zucchini.

4. Pour the wet ingredients into the dry and mix to combine.

5. Press the dough firmly into the loaf pan, and bake for 50 to 60 minutes, or until browned on the edges and a toothpick inserted in the center comes out clean.

6. Allow the bread to cool before slicing, or it might crumble.

7. Serve immediately, store in the refrigerator for up to 7 days, or slice and freeze for up to 3 months.

Minted Tahini Dip

A great alternative to hummus, for anyone who might be sensitive to beans or might be looking for a lower-carb alternative. I like to pair this dip with crudité, Seeded Crackers (page 193), or Purple Sweet Potato Fries (page 116).

MAKES ABOUT 2 CUPS

¼ cup chopped fresh mint

¼ cup chopped fresh parsley

¼ cup chopped fresh dill

1 garlic clove

1 cup tahini

Juice of 1 lemon

½ cup filtered water

1 tablespoon extra-virgin olive oil, divided

1 teaspoon sea salt

1. In a food processor, add the mint, parsley, dill, and garlic, and pulse until finely chopped.

2. Add the tahini, lemon juice, water, ½ tablespoon of the olive oil, and the salt, and pulse until smooth.

3. Serve immediately with a drizzle of the remaining olive oil, or store in an airtight container in the refrigerator for up to 1 week.

Golden Hummus

I love this hummus with crudité, Seeded Crackers (page 193), or as a big smear underneath your favorite salad or grain bowl. Golden beets add an earthy flavor and a creamier texture. Add a generous smear to the bottom of a meal-prep chicken or salmon bowl to make your meal feel like you ordered it at your favorite restaurant.

MAKES ABOUT 2 CUPS

2 golden beets, steamed and peeled

1 (15-ounce) can chickpeas, drained and rinsed

¼ cup tahini

⅓ cup extra-virgin olive oil

Zest and juice of 1 lemon

1 teaspoon ground cumin

½ teaspoon garlic powder

¼ teaspoon ground turmeric

1 teaspoon sea salt

¼ teaspoon freshly ground black pepper

In a food processor, combine the beets, chickpeas, tahini, olive oil, lemon zest, lemon juice, cumin, garlic powder, turmeric, salt, and pepper, and blend until smooth. Store in an airtight container in the refrigerator for up to 5 days.

Hard-Boiled Eggs with Dipping Salts

Get some interesting salt blends, like gomasio or everything bagel spice, to turn classic hard-boiled egg into an exciting savory snack.

MAKES 6 TO 12 EGGS

6 to 12 large eggs

Pinch of sea salt

Salt blend of choice (see Resources)

1. In a large saucepan, add the eggs and enough water to cover 1 to 2 inches above the eggs.

2. Add the salt to keep the eggs from cracking, and bring the water to a boil.

3. Once the water boils, turn off the heat and cover the saucepan, letting it sit for 10 to 12 minutes.

4. Strain the water and pour cold running water on top of the eggs. You can peel the eggs directly under the water, or store them in the shell in the refrigerator for up to 5 days.

5. When ready to eat, add some of the salt blend of choice to a plate and use for dipping the hard-boiled eggs.

Seeded Crackers

These crackers are shockingly easy to make and incredibly versatile. High in protein and fiber, they add that crunch your soups, salads, and dips have been craving!

MAKES ABOUT 2 CUPS OF CRACKERS

6 tablespoons ground flaxseeds

¼ cup white sesame seeds

¼ cup pumpkin seeds

¼ cup sunflower seeds

¼ cup hemp seeds

¼ teaspoon garlic powder

⅛ teaspoon ground turmeric

½ teaspoon sea salt

¼ teaspoon freshly ground black pepper

¾ cup filtered water

2 teaspoons extra-virgin olive oil

1. Preheat the oven to 350°F and line a baking sheet with parchment paper.

2. In a medium mixing bowl, add the flaxseeds, sesame seeds, pumpkin seeds, sunflower seeds, hemp seeds, garlic powder, turmeric, sea salt, and black pepper, and mix to combine.

3. Add the water, stir, and let sit for 5 to 10 minutes. During this time, the flaxseeds will absorb the water and the mixture will thicken.

4. Cut two pieces of parchment paper and coat each with a teaspoon of the olive oil. Using a rolling pin, roll the mixture between the sheets of parchment paper until it is about ⅛ inch thick.

5. Transfer the mixture to the prepared baking sheet and remove the top layer of parchment paper. Bake for 50 minutes, turning halfway through to ensure it cooks evenly.

6. Allow to cool before breaking up into crackers. They are best eaten fresh, but you can store them in an airtight container in the pantry for up to 5 days.

Crispy Smoked Paprika Chickpeas

Paprika, also known as pimenton, is a powerhouse spice both in flavor and nutrient content. It has seven times as much vitamin C as an orange and nine times more than a tomato! Smoked paprika has an intensely rich and smoky flavor that adds life to simple chickpeas. Enjoy as a crunchy, high-protein snack alongside some cut cucumbers and carrots, or as a soup or salad topper.

MAKES 1½ CUPS OF CHICKPEAS

1 (15-ounce) can chickpeas

1 tablespoon extra-virgin olive oil

1 teaspoon smoked paprika

1 teaspoon sea salt

1. Preheat the oven to 400°F and line a baking sheet with parchment paper.

2. Drain and rinse the chickpeas, then pat dry with a kitchen towel.

3. In a bowl, add the chickpeas and coat them with the olive oil, smoked paprika, and sea salt. Spread the chickpeas evenly across the prepared baking sheet, discarding any loose skins.

4. Bake for 25 to 30 minutes, or until the chickpeas are golden brown and crispy. Allow to dry, and store in an airtight container in the refrigerator for up to 5 days.

Spiced Date & Walnut Bites

The key to making this recipe is soft dates. It won't work if your dates are too hard or dry. If your dates don't have the soft, chewy texture we're looking for, just soak them in warm water for ten minutes before adding to the food processor.

MAKES 8 TO 10 BARS

2 cups soft pitted dates

2 cups raw walnuts

½ tablespoon ground cinnamon

1 teaspoon ground cardamom

Pinch of sea salt

1 cup unsweetened coconut flakes

1. In a food processor, combine the dates, walnuts, cinnamon, cardamom, and salt, and pulse until it's well combined and forms a ball. You may need to scrape the sides a few times, but some chunkier bits are ok.

2. In a bowl, add the coconut and set aside.

3. Lay some parchment paper down on a cutting board or your countertop, and using a rolling pin, roll out the date and walnut mixture. I like to roll into logs and cut into 1-inch bites, but you could also roll these into balls.

4. Once you have your desired shape, drop bites one by one into the coconut and coat completely.

5. Repeat with all pieces, and store in an airtight container in the refrigerator for up to 1 week.

Salted Chocolate Tart

Elegant, indulgent, and celebratory, this dessert hits the spot with just the slightest bit of unrefined sugars. It's almost too good to be true! Serve with Coconut Whipped Cream (page 205) and a sprig of mint for a fresh touch.

SERVES 8 TO 10

FOR THE CRUST
1½ cups almond flour

½ cup coconut flour

2 tablespoons coconut sugar

Pinch of sea salt

6 tablespoons melted ghee or coconut oil

FOR THE FILLING
1 (9-ounce) package of 70% cacao dark chocolate chips

1¼ cups full-fat unsweetened coconut milk

1 teaspoon vanilla extract

2 large eggs, beaten

Pinch of Maldon sea salt

Special equipment: You will need a 9-inch tart pan with a removable bottom for this recipe.

1. Make the crust. Preheat the oven to 350°F. In a bowl, combine the almond flour, coconut flour, coconut sugar, and salt, and mix thoroughly. Add the ghee, and use a fork or your hand to mix the ghee in until you can make a firm ball with the dough.

2. Add the crust to the tart pan, working the edges first.

3. Firmly press the remaining dough into the bottom of the pan. The dough should be half as thick on the bottom as it is on the edge.

4. Place the tart pan on a baking sheet and bake for 15 to 20 minutes, or until golden brown.

5. Remove the crust from the oven and let cool completely.

6. Make the filling. In a double boiler, add the chocolate, coconut milk, and vanilla extract, and cook, stirring with a spatula or wooden spoon, until melted and combined.

7. Allow the chocolate mixture to cool slightly, then add one spoonful of chocolate into the eggs to temper. This is to prevent the eggs from scrambling when you pour them into the hot chocolate mixture. Next, slowly add the eggs to the chocolate, stirring continuously to prevent the eggs from cooking.

8. Pour the filling into the tart pan and top with a generous pinch of Maldon sea salt. Place the tart pan on a baking sheet and bake for 30 minutes, or until it's almost firm (give it a little shake in the oven to test).

9. Remove the pan from the oven and allow the tart to cool completely before placing it in the refrigerator.

10. When you're ready to serve, push the bottom of the tart pan up to remove it from the pan.

Notes: You can bake your crust the day before, if you want to break the process up into two parts.

Spend a decent amount of time pressing the dough into the edges of the pan, making sure it is even throughout. A strong edge will form a strong crust that you can easily cut through, so don't skimp on that step.

Create a double boiler by heating water to a simmer in a pot and placing a heat-proof bowl on top. The bowl should rest nicely on top without touching the water.

POST-RESET RECIPE

Skillet Apple Crisp

This delicious, warming, and satisfying dessert has only 32 grams of added sugar total. Divide that into 6 portions, and that's less than 6 grams per serving. My general rule of thumb is to aim for less than 10 grams of sugar, and this treat certainly hits the mark.

SERVES 6

**4 Granny Smith apples,
   peeled, cored, and sliced
   into ½-inch wedges**

**1 teaspoon ground cinnamon,
   divided**

¼ teaspoon ground cardamom

1 teaspoon ground ginger

1 teaspoon lemon juice

1 tablespoon coconut sugar

¼ cup raisins

5 tablespoons water, divided

1 tablespoon ground flaxseeds

1½ cups rolled oats

1 cup almond flour

¼ teaspoon ground nutmeg

Pinch of sea salt

¼ cup chopped pecans

⅓ cup extra-virgin olive oil

**2 tablespoons brown rice
   syrup**

1. Preheat the oven to 350°F.

2. In a medium mixing bowl, add the apples, ½ teaspoon of the cinnamon, the cardamom, ginger, lemon juice, coconut sugar, and raisins. Mix to combine.

3. In a 10-inch cast-iron skillet, arrange the apples. Pour 2 tablespoons of the water over the apples.

4. In a small bowl, mix the flaxseeds and remaining 3 tablespoons of the water. Stir to combine and set aside.

5. In the same mixing bowl you had the apples in, add the oats, almond flour, nutmeg, sea salt, remaining ½ teaspoon of the cinnamon, and chopped pecans. Mix to combine.

6. Add the flaxseed mixture into the oat mixture, followed by the olive oil and brown rice syrup, and stir until fully incorporated.

7. Spread the oat mixture evenly over the apples and bake for 45 to 50 minutes, or until golden.

8. Serve warm. Goes great with a big scoop of vanilla ice cream (check the Resources section for my favorite brands).

POST-RESET RECIPE

SNACKS, SWEETS & BAKED GOODS

Salted Caramel Chocolate Fudge

When you just want a little chocolate indulgence, let this be your new go-to. With no added sugars, this is the perfect Reset treat as well.

MAKES ABOUT 2 CUPS

4 pitted Medjool dates

1 cup cashew butter

¼ cup coconut oil

¼ cup raw cacao powder

½ teaspoon vanilla extract

Pinch of Maldon sea salt

1. Line an 8-inch loaf pan with aluminum foil and set aside.

2. In a food processor, add the dates, and pulse until they form a paste.

3. Add the cashew butter, coconut oil, raw cacao powder, and vanilla extract to the food processor and mix until fully combined.

4. Pour the mixture into the loaf pan, give it a few taps on the countertop to even out, and top with a generous sprinkle of Maldon sea salt.

5. Place in the freezer for at least 1 hour to set, then cut into 1-inch squares and store in an airtight container in the refrigerator for 5 to 7 days or in the freezer for up to 3 months.

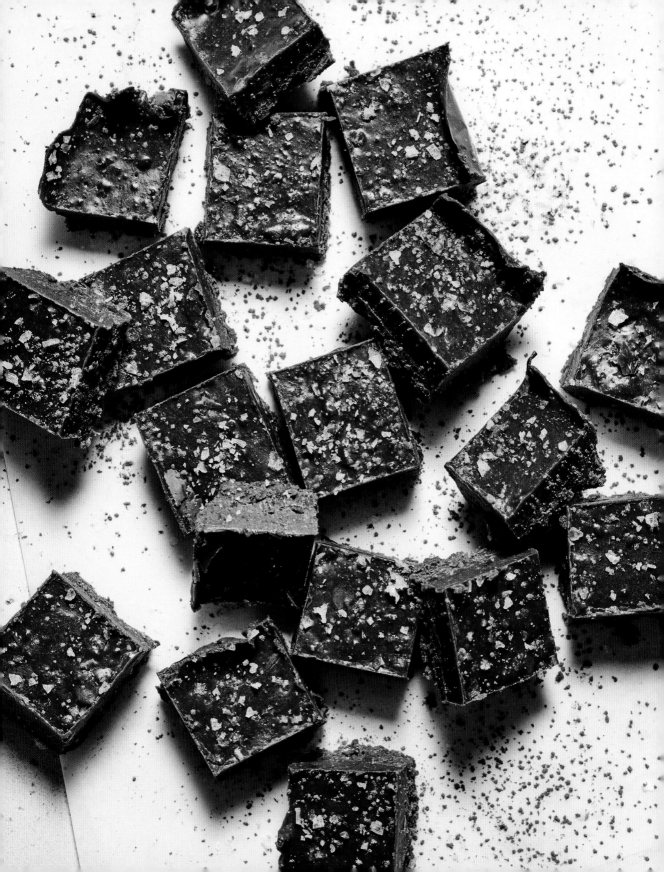

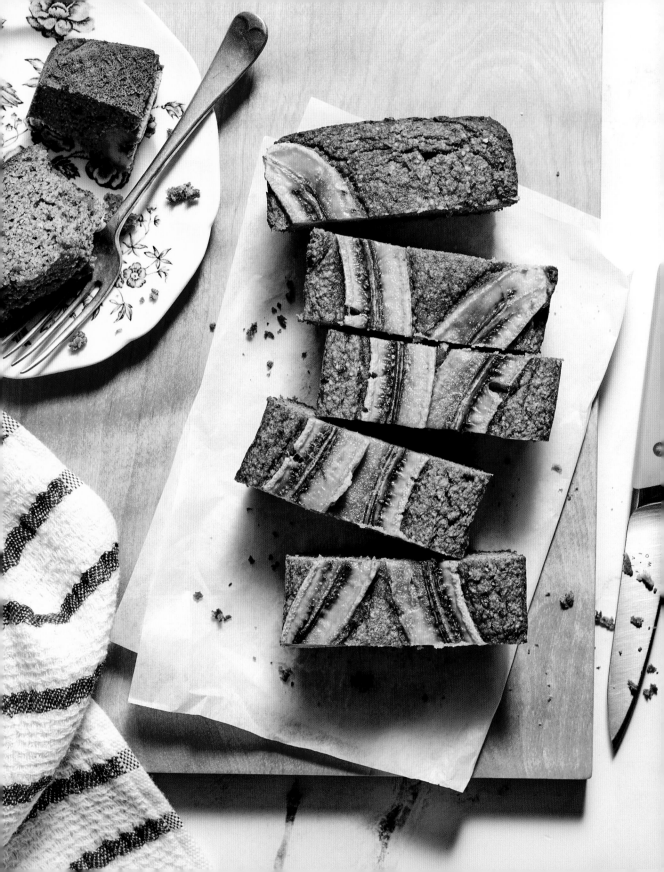

Banana Bread

I have tested and retested this recipe countless times with different types of sugar, and with no sugar at all, and landed on this. Originally the recipe had maple syrup, but I swapped the added sugar with two dates to make it Reset friendly. It still has a nice hint of sweetness, but without any added sugars.

SERVES 8

2 tablespoons coconut oil, plus more for greasing

3 bananas (2 overripe with brown spots, 1 fresh)

2 Medjool dates, pitted

2 large eggs

½ teaspoon vanilla extract

1 cup almond flour

¼ cup coconut flour

1 teaspoon baking soda

½ teaspoon ground cinnamon

½ teaspoon salt

1. Preheat the oven to 350°F and line a 9-inch loaf pan with parchment paper. I line the middle, letting the edges of the paper fall over the edge of the pan. Grease the sides of the pan with coconut oil for easy removal.

2. In a food processor, blend the ripe bananas with the dates. Pulse until fully combined.

3. Add the eggs, coconut oil, and vanilla extract, and mix thoroughly to combine.

4. In a separate bowl, mix the almond flour, coconut flour, baking soda, cinnamon, and salt.

5. Add the dry ingredients to the banana mixture, and mix until incorporated. Turn off the mixer and use a spatula to give the dough a good stir.

6. Place the dough in the prepared loaf pan. The dough is thick, so use a spatula to even it out.

7. Cut the fresh banana in half lengthwise and press it into the top of the dough, cut side up.

8. Bake for 30 minutes, or until a cake tester comes out clean.

9. When finished, use the edges of the parchment paper to lift the banana bread out of the pan. Store in the refrigerator for up to 5 days.

Chocolate-Avocado Mousse

Chocolate mousse will forever be my favorite dessert. I used to make the classic French version, but I have to say—health benefits aside—this version hits the spot for me and is ready in a fraction of the time. You cannot taste the avocado in this recipe, and it gives the mousse that signature creamy, silky texture. To make this Reset friendly, use stevia-sweetened chocolate chips (like Lily's), and monk fruit sweetener.

SERVES 4 TO 6

¼ cup dark chocolate chips

2 ripe avocados, peeled and pit removed

¼ cup raw cacao powder

½ teaspoon vanilla extract

¼ cup non-dairy milk of choice

¼ cup monk fruit sweetener, maple syrup, honey, or coconut sugar

Pinch of sea salt

Toppings: Cacao nibs, pumpkin seeds, and/or hemp seeds (optional)

Note: You can use a blender if you don't have a food processor, but it's a little more arduous and requires extra patience and scraping down the sides.

1. In a double boiler, melt the chocolate (see Note page 196).

2. Place the melted chocolate, avocados, raw cacao powder, vanilla extract, non-dairy milk, sweetener, and sea salt in a food processor, and pulse until fully combined. You may need to pause and scrape down the sides a few times to avoid any avocado chucks and ensure a creamy texture.

3. Portion the mousse into four to 6 individual airtight containers and add toppings, if using. The mousse will last in the refrigerator for about 3 days.

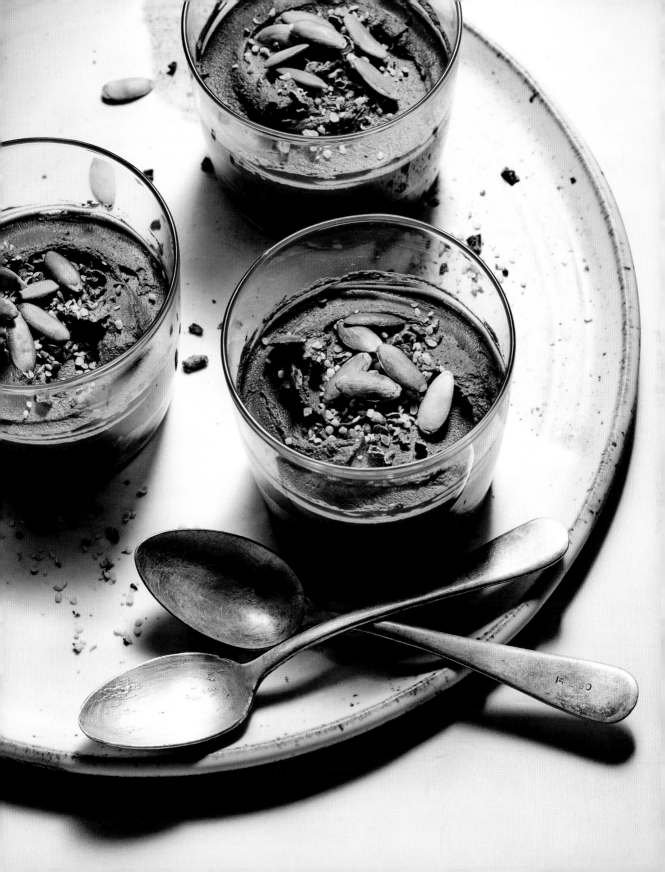

Coconut Macaroons

I like to keep these low-sugar, high-protein treats in the fridge as an easy dessert. You can always skip the chocolate dip if you prefer a plain macaroon.

MAKES 12 MACAROONS

4 large egg whites

2 tablespoons maple syrup

1 teaspoon vanilla extract

3 cups unsweetened shredded coconut

Pinch of sea salt

½ cup dark chocolate chips (optional)

1. Preheat the oven to 350°F and line a baking sheet with parchment paper.

2. Using a stand mixer, whisk together the egg whites, maple syrup, and vanilla extract until fully incorporated.

3. Add the shredded coconut and sea salt. Mix until fully combined.

4. Using an ice cream scoop or a large spoon, portion out 12 balls of the coconut mixture onto the prepared baking sheet.

5. Bake for 20 to 22 minutes, or until browned. Let cool completely.

6. Meanwhile, melt chocolate chips over a double boiler (see Note page 000). Dip each cooled macaroon into the melted chocolate and place them back on the baking sheet. Once all macaroons have been dipped, you can drizzle extra chocolate on top, if desired.

7. Place the macaroons in the freezer to set for at least 20 minutes.

8. Store in an airtight container in the refrigerator for up to 7 days or in the freezer for up to 3 months.

Grilled Peaches with Coconut Whipped Cream

A perfectly ripe peach should be on everyone's summer bucket list. During peak stone-fruit season, I'm always looking for ways to enjoy this amazing fruit, and if this is your first time grilling a peach, it certainly won't the be last. This recipe is Reset friendly, but if you want to take up it a notch post-Reset, marinate your peaches in whiskey for an hour before grilling them.

SERVES 4

Coconut cream from
    1 (13.5-ounce) can organic,
    unsweetened full-fat
    coconut milk, refrigerated
    overnight (see Note)

½ teaspoon vanilla extract or
    fresh vanilla

2 ripe peaches

1 tablespoon extra-virgin
    olive oil

4 sprigs fresh mint

1. Before making your whipped cream, place the bowl and beater from a stand mixer or the beaters from a handheld mixer in the freezer for 10 minutes to make sure everything is nice and cold.

2. Whip the coconut cream and vanilla extract on high for a few minutes, or until it thickens. Transfer the whipped cream to an airtight container and store in the refrigerator until ready to consume.

3. When ready to serve, halve the peaches, remove the pits, and brush with the olive oil. Grill cut side down for 3 to 4 minutes, then rotate 90 degrees and grill for another 3 minutes.

4. To serve, place a peach half, cut side up, on a plate. Top with a large spoonful of the coconut whipped cream and a sprig of mint.

Notes: When you open the coconut milk, a thick cream should have formed separate from a clear(ish) liquid. The cream is what we want. Scoop into a bowl and reserve the liquid; you can drink it or add to a smoothie; it's essentially coconut water.

You can also enjoy this whipped cream with fresh berries , the Salted Chocolate Tart (page 196), or the Skillet Apple Crisp (page 197).

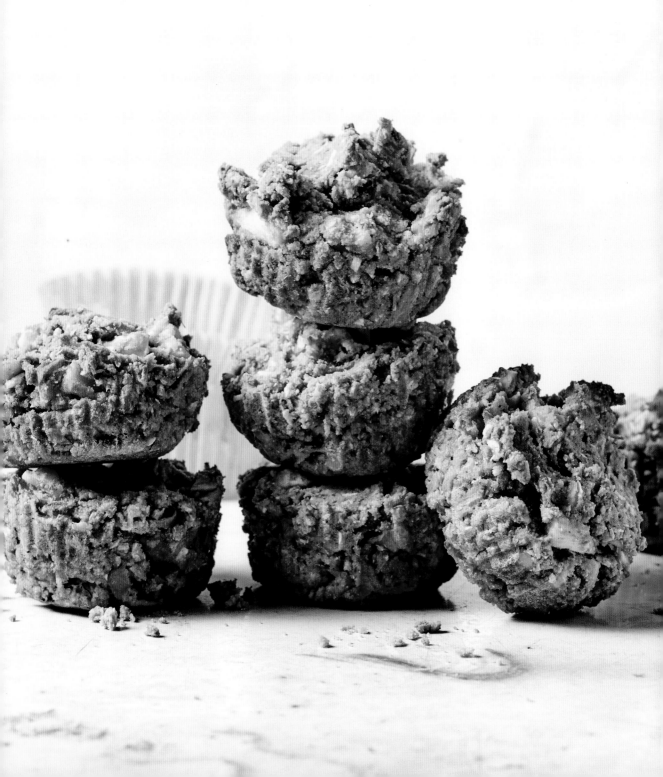

Carrot-Apple Snack Muffins

Sometimes you just need a muffin, but most baked goods are full of sugar and gluten, and not incredibly nutrient-dense. These Carrot-Apple Snack Muffins are sweetened only with a banana and dried apple slices, and they are the perfect afternoon or morning treat alongside a cup of tea.

MAKES 10 TO 12 MUFFINS

1 ripe banana

2 large eggs

1 heaping cup grated carrots

2 cups almond flour

½ cup shredded coconut flakes

1 teaspoon baking soda

1 teaspoon baking powder

1 teaspoon ground cinnamon

½ teaspoon ground ginger

½ teaspoon sea salt

½ cup walnuts, roughly chopped

½ cup dried apples, roughly chopped about the same size of the walnuts

1. Preheat the oven to 350°F and line a muffin tin with liners.

2. In a medium bowl, mash the banana, then whisk in the eggs until creamy. Stir in the grated carrots.

3. In a separate bowl, whisk together the almond flour, coconut flakes, baking soda, baking powder, cinnamon, ginger, and salt.

4. Use a spatula to fold the dry ingredients into the wet, and continue to mix until fully incorporated. Mix in the walnuts and dried apples.

5. Evenly distribute the muffin batter in the muffin tin, and bake for 22 to 25 minutes, or until a toothpick comes out clean.

6. Store in an airtight container in the refrigerator for up to 5 days.

Elevated Pantry Essentials

The goal of meal prepping is to stock your refrigerator and pantry with pre-prepared foods so you can throw a meal together in less than ten minutes.

As convenient as meal prep might be, it can quickly get boring and monotonous. That's where these pantry essentials come in handy. When you have flavorful, high-quality, and nutrient-dense pantry items, you can make even the simplest and quickest of meals much more exciting.

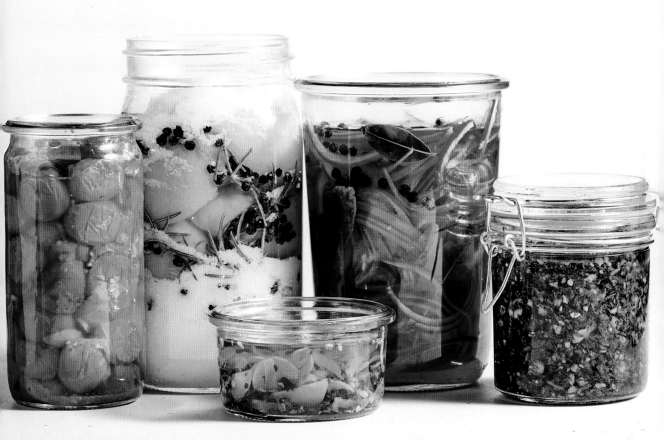

Pickled Red Onions

Keep a jar of these in your refrigerator to add that hint of zing to your salads, sandwiches, and bowls. An easy way to make a throw-together dish feel like restaurant quality.

MAKES ABOUT 1½ CUPS

1 medium red onion

2 bay leaves

½ tablespoon black peppercorns

½ cup red wine vinegar, plus more as needed

½ cup water

2 teaspoons sea salt

1. Use a mandoline or a sharp knife to thinly slice the red onion, and place in a glass jar with a tight-fitting lid. Add the bay leaves and peppercorns.

2. In a bowl, combine the red wine vinegar, water, and salt, whisking until the salt dissolves.

3. Pour the liquid in the jar to cover the onions. If the onions are not completely covered, add more vinegar.

4. Let the onions sit for at least 1 hour before eating, and store in the refrigerator for up to 1 week.

Tomato Confit

There are many ways to use tomato confit in everyday cooking, especially on The Reset. It's a great addition to pastas, soups, salads, or grain bowls, and makes an excellent topping for simply cooked proteins.

MAKES ABOUT 1½ CUPS

1 pound cherry tomatoes, on or off the vine

2 to 3 garlic cloves, sliced

¼ cup extra-virgin olive oil, plus more as needed

1 fresh rosemary sprig

Sea salt, to taste

1. Preheat the oven to 275°F.

2. In a large baking dish, place the tomatoes and garlic all in one row.

3. Cover the tomatoes with the olive oil, add the rosemary sprig, and season with the salt.

4. Bake for 90 minutes, or until the tomatoes have popped and are slightly toasted. Remove the tomatoes from the oven and allow them to cool.

5. Store the tomatoes in an airtight container in the refrigerator covered with the cooking olive oil. If the olive oil doesn't cover the tomatoes completely, add more.

6. Keep the confit in the refrigerator for up to 2 weeks.

Chocolate-Hazelnut Spread

I am particular about hazelnuts. I don't like them with everything, but they are magical paired with chocolate. Hazelnuts are also an excellent source of plant-based proteins and healthy fats—including those coveted omega-3s. Spread this all over a slice of Nut & Seed Protein Bread (page 191) for an incredibly satisfying snack high in protein, fiber, and healthy fats.

MAKES ABOUT 2 CUPS

2 cups hazelnuts

1 tablespoon avocado oil

⅓ cup raw cacao powder

¼ to ⅓ cup sweetener of choice (Use monk fruit to make this sugar free and Reset friendly.)

Pinch of sea salt

1. Preheat the oven to 350°F and line a baking sheet with parchment paper.

2. Spread the hazelnuts across the baking sheet and bake for 15 to 20 minutes, or until lightly toasted and fragrant.

3. Take the hazelnuts out of the oven and allow them to cool. Place the hazelnuts in a kitchen towel and rub the hazelnut skins off. The more skin you can get off, the smoother your dip will be, but it doesn't have to be perfect.

4. In a food processor or high-speed blender, add the hazelnuts and blend until smooth and the consistency of nut butter. This could take a while depending on the strength of your food processor or blender, so be patient and scrape the sides down as necessary.

5. Add the avocado oil, cacao powder, sweetener, and sea salt. Blend for an additional minute, or until fully incorporated.

6. Store in an airtight container in the refrigerator for up to 3 weeks. Yes, this means it should last for the duration of your Reset.

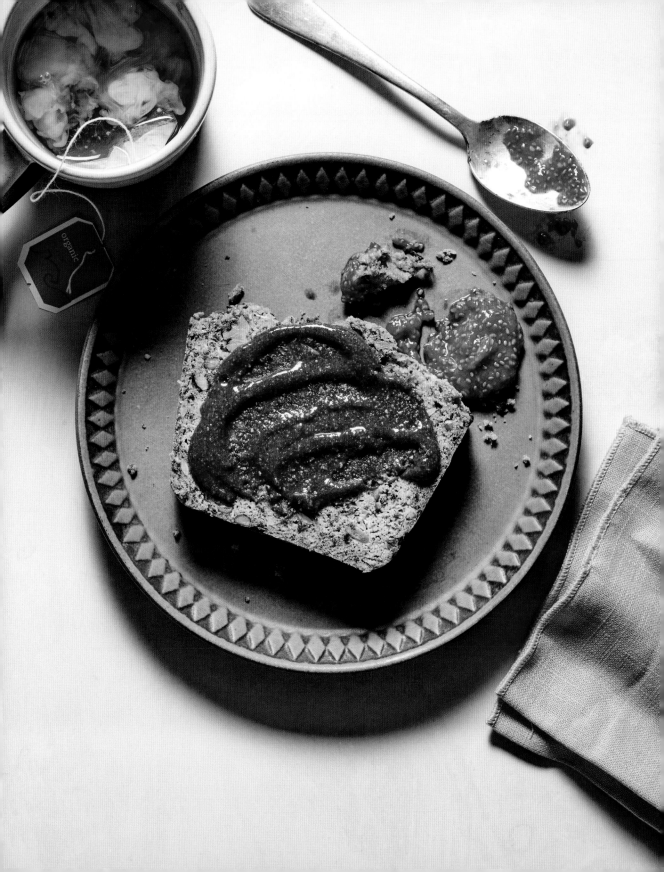

Raspberry-Chia Jam

Commercial jams are full of added sugars. Not only is this jam sweetened with just fruit, but it is also paired with protein, fiber, and fat-rich chia seeds to balance out any blood sugar spikes. Spread on a slice of Nut & Seed Protein Bread (page 191) or a brown rice cake with almond butter for a satisfying snack.

MAKES ABOUT 1 CUP

2 cups raspberries, frozen or fresh

2 tablespoons white chia seeds

2 tablespoons filtered water

Squeeze of lemon juice

In a blender, combine the raspberries, chia seeds, water, and lemon juice, and blend until well combined, about 30 seconds. Store in an airtight container in the refrigerator for up to 1 week.

Crispy Shallots & Shallot Olive Oil

These crispy shallots are hard to resist, and you'll want to use them immediately, but this shallot oil is a side effect that your pantry needs. On particularly busy days, I will make myself scrambled eggs with a side of greens dressed with this shallot oil, lemon juice, and sea salt for lunch. It truly feels like I've ordered an omelet in Paris, not rushed to make lunch in five minutes.

MAKES 1 CUP CRISPY SHALLOTS PLUS 1 CUP SHALLOT OLIVE OIL

3 medium shallots, thinly sliced

Extra-virgin olive oil

1 to 2 teaspoons sea salt

1. Cover a plate with a paper towel and set aside.

2. In a large skillet, place the shallots and enough olive oil to cover them completely. Turn heat to low and cook, stirring frequently, until browned, 20 to 25 minutes. The shallots should be a dark brown (not burnt, but dark), otherwise they will not get crispy.

3. Use a fork or a slotted spoon to transfer the shallots to the prepared plate. Season immediately with salt. They will get crispy as they dry.

4. Store the shallot-infused olive oil in an airtight glass container at room temperature for up to 7 days.

Garlic Chili Oil

Whenever I make this garlic chili oil, I find myself wanting to put it on absolutely everything, from pastas, soups, sautéed greens, and more. The combination of vitamin C–rich chili and garlic also makes this condiment a great immune booster.

MAKES ABOUT ½ CUP

½ cup extra-virgin olive oil

10 garlic cloves, thinly sliced

2 tablespoons red pepper flakes

1. In a small saucepan, heat the olive oil over medium heat.

2. Add the garlic and cook, stirring constantly, for 3 to 5 minutes, or until lightly browned but not burnt. Reduce the heat if it looks like the garlic is getting too brown.

3. Turn off the heat and stir in the red pepper flakes.

4. Cool and transfer the mixture to an airtight container. Store in the refrigerator for 1 week. If you want the oil to last longer, remove the garlic cloves and store the oil in an airtight container at room temperature.

Preserved Lemons

It takes three whole months for your preserved lemons to be ready to cook with, but it's well worth the time investment. Use these in any recipe that calls for lemon or lemon zest to add a bright, salty, and umami-rich citrus flavor to the dish. A very convenient (and delicious) swap when you've run out of lemons.

MAKES 9 TO 10 PRESERVED LEMONS

9 to 10 organic lemons

Sea salt

1 tablespoon black peppercorns

1 sprig fresh rosemary

1. Make an X cut from the top of 4 to 5 lemons, almost quartering them, but leaving about half on the bottom to keep the lemon intact.

2. Rub a generous amount of salt inside each lemon.

3. In the bottom of a medium jam jar, add a layer of salt. Press the lemons into the jar, one by one, sprinkling a layer of salt over each lemon.

4. Nestle the black peppercorns and rosemary sprig in the jar with the lemons. Repeat until all lemons are snugly in the jar, separating any lemons that don't fit.

5. Juice the remaining lemons into the jar until the lemons are completely submerged in liquid.

6. Close the jar and leave in your pantry to ripen at room temperature. Make sure to give the jar a good shake each day for 4 weeks, or until the rinds are tender.

7. Once the lemons are preserved, store them in the jar in the refrigerator until ready to use.

8. To use, remove a piece of lemon from the jar and rinse off the salt. The rind is great raw or as a finishing flavor to a cooked dish.

9. Store the preserved lemons in the refrigerator for up to 1 year.

Brazil Nut Romesco

Dietary diversity is important for getting more nutrition out of the foods you eat, and I hope these recipes encourage you to switch things up a little bit. Enter Brazil nuts: Full of minerals like selenium (which is great for the thyroid), magnesium, and zinc; antioxidants like vitamin E; protein; monounsaturated fats; and fiber, these nuts are a powerhouse and lend a smooth, buttery texture to this recipe. Serve alongside grilled proteins and vegetables, as a dip, or with an appetizer board.

MAKES ABOUT 2 CUPS

1 jar roasted red peppers, drained

½ cup sun-dried tomatoes

½ cup Brazil nuts

½ cup extra-virgin olive oil, plus more as needed

1 garlic clove

1 teaspoon smoked paprika

½ teaspoon cayenne pepper

1 teaspoon sea salt

1. In a high-speed blender or food processor, add the roasted peppers, sun-dried tomatoes, Brazil nuts, olive oil, garlic, paprika, cayenne, and salt, and blend until smooth. If the mixture gets to thick, add more olive oil, 1 tablespoon at a time.

2. Store the romesco in an airtight container in the refrigerator for up to 7 days.

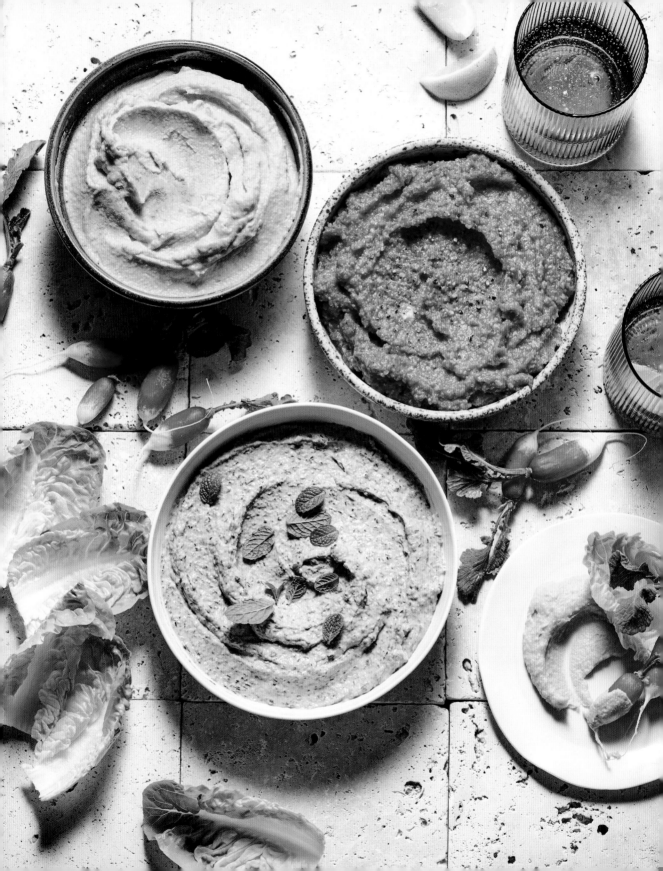

Pistachio Pistou

Pistou is like a French pesto. Instead of a basil base, this sauce uses a variety of herbs, like parsley and dill, in addition to basil. I like to keep it a little chunky and add to roasted meats or as a garnish to soups. It pairs especially well with the Roasted Cauliflower & Garlic (page 186) and White Bean & Leek (page 178) soups.

MAKES ABOUT 1 CUP

½ cup shelled pistachios

1 cup fresh basil leaves

1 cup fresh parsley leaves

1 cup fresh dill

1 garlic clove

¼ teaspoon red pepper flakes

Zest of 1 lemon

1 tablespoon lemon juice

½ cup extra-virgin olive oil

Sea salt, to taste

1. In a food processor, add the pistachios, basil, parsley, dill, garlic, red pepper flakes, lemon zest, lemon juice, olive oil, and salt, and pulse lightly to combine.

2. Store in an airtight container in the refrigerator for up to 5 days.

Curried Coconut Sauce

This is the sauce you put on your food when you're not sure what to make. It takes just a few minutes to whip up and will electrify even the most mundane of meals.

MAKES ABOUT 1 CUP

1 cup full-fat, unsweetened coconut milk

1 teaspoon curry powder

½ tablespoon minced garlic

½ tablespoon minced fresh ginger

Pinch of sea salt

Squeeze of lime juice

1. In a small saucepan, add the coconut milk and heat over low-medium heat.

2. Add the curry powder, minced garlic, minced ginger, and salt, and stir with a wooden spoon until it thickens a little, 3 to 5 minutes.

3. Add in a squeeze of lime juice, and serve with your favorite protein or vegetables, or store in an airtight container in the refrigerator for up to 5 days.

Tarragon Salsa Verde

Tarragon is a wildly underrated herb. It has a delicate, peppery anise taste that pairs really well with chicken and white fish. As with all herbs, tarragon also boasts a litany of health benefits. It is known for promoting good digestion, reducing inflammation and blood sugar, and improving sleep patterns.

MAKES ABOUT 1 CUP

½ cup fresh tarragon

1 cup fresh parsley

1 medium shallot

1 garlic clove

Zest and juice of one lemon

1 tablespoon capers, drained

1 teaspoon Dijon mustard

¾ cup extra-virgin olive oil

Sea salt and freshly ground black pepper, to taste

Note: If you don't have a food processor, you can finely chop these ingredients with a knife and add them together.

1. In a food processor, add the tarragon, parsley, shallot, garlic, lemon zest, and capers to a food processor, and pulse until finely chopped but not pureed.

2. In a small bowl, whisk together the lemon juice, mustard, and olive oil. Add to the food processor, and pulse until fully combined.

3. Taste and season with salt and pepper as desired.

4. Store in an airtight container in the refrigerator for up to 7 days.

Nut & Seed Milks

Making nut milks at home is easier than you think, and always the most nutritious option when it comes to dairy alternatives.

Fresh nut and seed milks are higher in healthy fats than most commercial milks, so if you're using in a smoothie, you can cut down on the fat content. Here are few recipes to get you started.

Classic Almond Milk

This is the classic formula for almond milk, and it never disappoints. I especially love the froth on the milk when it's fresh from the blender. Excellent for all your caffeinated and non-caffeinated latte creations, and (of course) smoothies.

MAKES 4 CUPS

1 cup raw almonds, soaked overnight in filtered water

4 cups filtered water

½ teaspoon vanilla extract

Pinch of sea salt

1. Drain the almonds and add them to a high-speed blender along with the water, vanilla extract, and sea salt.

2. Blend on high until white in color, about 60 seconds.

3. Strain through a nut milk bag into a mixing bowl with a pour spout. Squeeze the bag until you get out as much milk as possible.

4. Store in an airtight container in the refrigerator for up to 5 days.

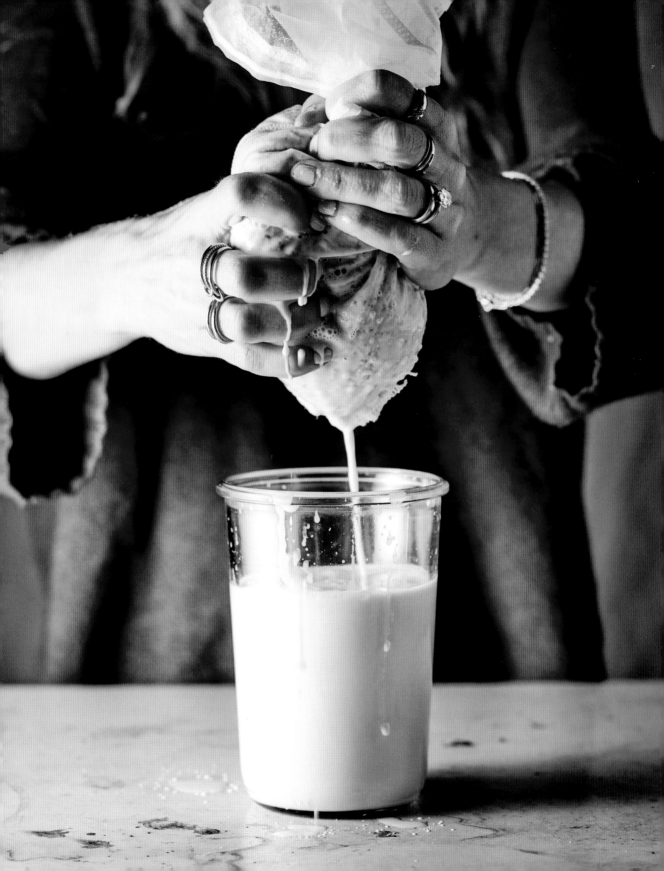

Black Sesame–Coconut Milk

Black sesame seeds are a great source of plant-based protein, calcium, magnesium, zinc, antioxidants, and B-vitamins. I love this nut-free, non-dairy milk option, and often make this for my son. He loves the taste, and I love the nutrition content (and that you don't have to remember to soak your seeds overnight—this only applies to nuts!).

MAKES 4 CUPS

4 cups filtered water

1 cup unsweetened coconut flakes

¼ cup black sesame seeds

½ teaspoon vanilla extract

Pinch of sea salt

1. In a high-speed blender, combine the water, coconut flakes, black sesame seeds, vanilla extract, and salt, and blend until smooth, about 1 minute.

2. Strain through a nut milk bag into a mixing bowl with a pour spout, and store in an airtight container in the refrigerator for 3 to 5 days.

Walnut-Cinnamon Milk

Cinnamon gives this creamy milk a warm, nutty flavor and helps regulate your blood sugar levels, and walnuts are an excellent source of anti-inflammatory omega-3 fatty acids. Use in your morning coffee, with granola, in a smoothie, or drink on its own.

MAKES 4 CUPS

1 cup walnuts

4 cups filtered water, plus extra for soaking

1 teaspoon ground cinnamon

1 teaspoon vanilla extract

Pinch of sea salt

1. Soak the walnuts in filtered water overnight.

2. Drain the walnuts, and add them to a high-speed blender with the 4 cups of water, cinnamon, vanilla extract, and sea salt.

3. Blend on high for 2 minutes. Pour through a nut milk bag or cheesecloth into a mixing bowl with a pour spout, then transfer to an airtight container and store in the refrigerator for 3 to 5 days.

Hydration
Station

Drinking water might sound like the oldest trick in the book, but despite its obvious nature, so many people do not drink enough water.

If you struggle to get your hydration in or find yourself getting bored of plain water, make it more exciting by adding natural flavorings, like fruits, vegetables, and herbs.

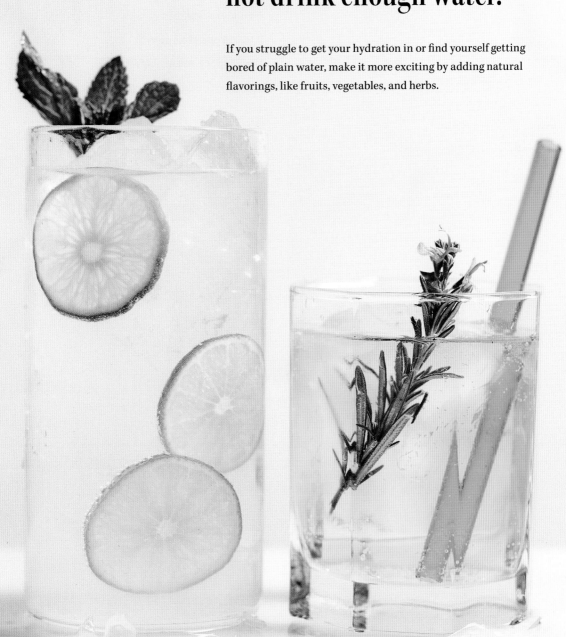

My Favorite Mocktail

Sometimes it feels good to have "something" at the end of the day. Instead of a nightly cocktail or glass of wine, try this mocktail recipe; it's refreshing and interesting to drink. Bitters are concentrations of herbs, spices, fruits, and botanicals that add flavor and are known to help with digestion. While they are distilled in alcohol, they are considered nonalcoholic because they are only consumed in miniscule drops, which makes the alcohol content undetectable.

MAKES 1 DRINK

8 ounces sparkling water

5 to 8 dashes bitters

Squeeze of lime juice

1 rosemary sprig (for garnish)

In a cocktail glass with ice, add the sparkling water and bitters. Stir to combine, then top with fresh lime juice and garnish with a rosemary sprig. Serve immediately.

Chlorophyll Lemonade

Chlorophyll is a natural compound found in green plants that gives them their signature hue and offer many health benefits. It is a wonderful antioxidant and potent anti-inflammatory agent and has also been dubbed nature's deodorant for helping control body odors.

MAKES 1 DRINK

8 ounces water

2 to 4 drops chlorophyll

1 tablespoon lemon juice

1 to 2 drops liquid stevia (optional)

In a glass (with or without ice), add the water, chlorophyll, lemon juice, and liquid stevia (if using), and stir to combine. Serve immediately.

Cinnamon Water

Cinnamon is a powerful spice that is known for balancing blood sugar levels. I have always found it interesting that we intuitively put cinnamon on sweets; a little trick from nature.

SERVES 3 TO 4

2 cinnamon sticks

6 cups water

1. In a large pot, add the cinnamon sticks and cover with the water.

2. Bring the mixture to a boil, then turn off the heat and allow it to cool.

3. Once cool, transfer the cinnamon water to an airtight container, and store it on the counter or in the refrigerator for up to 5 days.

Mint Mojito Electrolyte

Electrolytes are minerals that help maintain the balance of fluids in the body. They include sodium, potassium, magnesium, and calcium. Electrolyte drinks are hydrating and energizing, and generally include one or more of the aforementioned minerals. This drink gets a hint of potassium and magnesium from the lime juice, plus a healthy serving of salt.

MAKES 1 DRINK

10 fresh mint leaves

Juice of 1 lime

½ teaspoon pink Himalaya salt

⅛ teaspoon monk fruit sugar

2 cups sparkling water

1. In a large liquid measuring cup, add the mint leaves and lime juice. Break up the mint leaves a little using the back of a spoon until it gets really fragrant.

2. Add the salt and sugar, and whisk to combine.

3. Pour in the sparkling water, strain through a fine-mesh sieve, and serve over ice.

Resources

Pantry

Below is a list of brands and products that are my go-tos when I'm shopping for pantry staples. Your local grocer and farmers' market likely have small-batch products of equal quality, so don't worry if you can't find the exact brands or products listed. Once you start looking around, you will be able to find items that work for your shopping needs and budget!

Olive Oil

Brightland brightland.co

California Olive Ranch californiaoliveranch.com

Thrive Market thrivemarket.com

Condiments, Salad Dressings, & Marinades

Primal Kitchen primalkitchen.com

Chosen Foods chosenfoods.com

Dark Horse Organic darkhorseorganic.com

Coconut Amino Acids
nutiva.com

Bragg bragg.com

Sauerkraut store.edenfoods.com

Protein Powder

Primal Kitchen primalkitchen.com

Vital Proteins vitalproteins.com

Sunwarrior sunwarrior.com

Sakara Protein and Greens sakara.com

Ora So Lean and So Clean ora.organic

Pasta & Legumes

Tolerant Foods tolerantfoods.com

Banza eatbanza.com

Cappello's cappellos.com

Explore Cuisine explorecuisine.com

Shiratake Noodles miraclenoodle.com

Eden Foods store.edenfoods.com

Bread & Tortillas

Mikey's English Muffins eatmikeys.com

Young Kobra youngkobras.com

Omega Buns omegabun.com

Grindstone Bakery grindstonebakery.com

Base Culture baseculture.com

Siete Family Foods sietefoods.com

Chips, Crackers, & Snack Foods

Mary's Gone Crackers marysgonecrackers.com

Simple Mills simplemills.com

Siete Family Foods sietefoods.com

Lesser Evil lesserevil.com

Le Pain des Fleurs lepaindesfleurs.us

Protein Bars

REDD reddbar.com

Kalumi Beauty Food kalumibeauty.com

Sakara Super Bars sakara.com

Chocolate & Sweet Treats

Hu Kitchen hukitchen.com

Lily's Chocolate lilys.com

Eating Evolved eatingevolved.com

Addictive Wellness addictivewellness.com

Alter Eco Truffles alterecofoods.com

Fine and Raw fineandraw.com

Honey Mama's honeymamas.com

Dream Pops dreampops.com

Nada Moo nadamoo.com

Cereal

Three Wishes threewishescereal.com
Lovebird lovebirdfoods.com

Salts, Spices, & Seasonings

Diaspora diasporaco.com
Burlap and Barrell burlapandbarrel.com
Jennifer Fisher Universal Salt
jenniferfisherjewelry.com
Momofuku Seasoned Salts shop.momofuku.com
New York Shuk nyshuk.com
Eden Foods Gomasio store.edenfoods.com
Maldon Sea Salt maldonsalt.com

Specialty Food Products

Cap Beauty Coconut Butter capbeauty.com
Roe Caviar roecaviar.com
Miyoko's Creamery miyokos.com
Seed + Mill Tahini seedandmill.com
Harissa nyshuk.com

Online Groceries & Butchers

Thrive Market thrivemarket.com
Misfits Market misfitsmarket.com
Imperfect Foods imperfectfoods.com
Farmbox Direct farmboxdirect.com
Butcher Box butcherbox.com
Patagonia Provisions patagoniaprovisions.com

Prepared & Frozen Foods

Primal Kitchen primalkitchen.com
Caulipower Foods eatcaulipower.com
Good Stock Soups goodstocksoups.com
Daily Harvest daily-harvest.com

Drinks

Coffee Alternatives

Dandy Blend dandyblend.com
MUD\WTR mudwtr.com
Teeccino teeccino.com
Wooden Spoon Herbs Herbal Coffee woodenspoonherbs.com
Blue Lotus Chai bluelotuschai.com
Golde golde.co

Refreshments

Drink Sound drinksound.com
Guayakí Yerba Mate guayaki.com
Gerolsteiner Mineral Sparkling Water
gerolsteiner.de
Bragg ACV Refreshers bragg.com
Hoplark HopTea hoplark.com
HOP WTR hopwtr.com
Kin Euphorics kineuphorics.com
Nixie drinknixie.com
Liquid Death liquiddeath.com
LMNT Electrolyte drinklmnt.com

Tea

Bellocq Tea bellocqtea.com
Pique Tea piquelife.com
Organic India organicindisusa.com
Rishi Tea rishi-tea.com
House of Waris Botanicals houseofwaris.com
Anima Mundi animamundiherbals.com

Non-Dairy Milks

Malibu Mylk malibumylk.com
Malk Organics malkorganics.com
New Barn Organics newbarnorganics.com
Three Trees Organics threetrees.com

Supplements & Herbal/ Botanical Remedies

Probiotics

Seed seed.com

Klaire Labs klaire.com

Just Thrive Health justthrivehealth.com

Multivitamins

Metagenics metagneics.com

Thorne thorne.com

Klaire Labs klaire.com

Pure Encapsulations pureencapsulations.com

Sleep Support & Stress Management

Moon Juice Magnesi-om moonjuice.com

Hilma Sleep Support hilma.co

Anima Mundi Lucid Dreaming Tonic animamundiherbals.com

Innate Response Formulas Adrenal Response innateresponse.com

Kiva Sleep Cannabis-Infused Botanical Mints kivaconfections.com

Digestive Relief

Arrae Bloat arrae.com

Hilma Upset Stomach Relief hilma.co

Genexa Antacid genexa.com

Immune & Antioxidant Support

LivOn Labs Liposomal Vitamin C livonlabs.com

Anima Mundi Soma Elixir animamundiherbals.com

Source Naturals Wellness Formula sourcenaturals.com

Quicksilver Scientific Liposomal Glutathione quicksilverscientific.com

NSAID Alternative

Hilma Tension Relief hilma.co

Menstrual Wellness

Elix elixhealing.com

Kitchen & Home

Kitchen Appliances & Cooking Tools

Beast Health Blender thebeast.com

Breville Control Grip Immersion Blender breville.com

VitaClay Pressure Cooker vitaclaychef.com

Balmuda Toaster Oven us.balmuda.com

Kitchen Aid Stand Mixer kitchenaid.com

Cuisinart Food Processor cuisinart.com

Staub zwilling.com/us/staub/

Le Creuset lecreuset.com

Greenpan greenpan.us

Our Place fromourplace.com

Nordic Ware nordicware.com

Nut Milk Bag amazon.com

Tabletop & Home

Heath Ceramics heathceramics.com

Bitossi Home bitossihome.it

Roman and Williams Guild rwguild.com

Humble Ceramics humbleceramics.com

Nickey Kehoe nickeykehoe.com

Hawkins hawkinsnewyork.com

Shoppe Amber Interiors shoppe.amberinteriors.com

Vitruvi Diffuser vitruvi.com

Cinnamon Projects cinnamonprojects.com

Molekule Home Air Purifier molekule.com

Parachute Home parachutehome.com

Flamingo Estate flamingoestate.com

Berkey Water Filter berkeyfilters.com

Cleaning Products

Seventh Generation seventhgeneration.com

Branch Basics branchbasics.com

Dr. Bronners drbronner.com

Ecover us.ecover.com

Koala Eco koala.eco

Beauty
Face & Body
Linne Botanicals linnebotanicals.com

De Mamiel demamiel.com

Marie Veronique marieveronique.com

Kari Gran karigran.com

Osea Malibu oseamalibu.com

Wildling wildling.com

Oui the People ouithepeople.com

Nécessaire necessaire.com

goop goop.com

Makeup
Saie Beauty saiehello.com

Jones Road jonesroadbeauty.com

Westman Atelier westman-atelier.com

RMS rmsbeauty.com

Kosas kosas.com

Ilia iliabeauty.com

Hair Care
Playa playabeauty.com

Crown Affair crownaffair.com

Prose prose.com

Olaplex olaplex.com

Briogeo briogeohair.com

Fitness at Home
The Sculpt Society thesculptsociety.com

obé fitness obefitness.com

Peloton onepeloton.com

Lia Bartha Pilates bmethod.com

Tracy Anderson Method tracyanderson.com

Bulldog Yoga bulldogonline.com

Corepower Yoga corepoweryoga.com

Bala shopbala.com

Wearable Wellness Technology
Continuous Glucose Monitoring: Levels Health levelshealth.com

Sleep Tracker: Oura Ring ouraring.com

Infrared Sauna Blanket higherdose.com

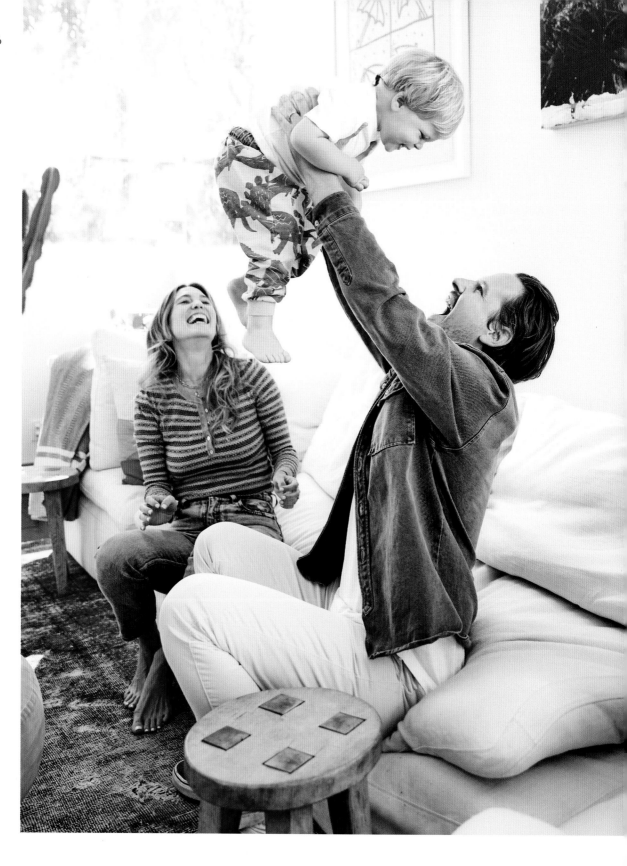

Acknowledgments

First and foremost, I want to thank my mom and dad for their continual enthusiasm and support even when I wanted to move to far flung, unfamiliar places and do crazy things. You've always taken my lead and given me the space to develop my own passions and skills. To my husband, Jamie, and my son, Ozzie, for bringing me so much joy, possibility, and constant laughs, giving me true purpose, trying all the food I cook, and being the best models for the pictures in this book. I love you both endlessly.

Foodwise would not have been possible without my agent, Rica Allannic. Thank you for understanding my vision and guiding me through the process of writing my first book. To Anja Schmidt for giving me a chance, and to Leah Miller for helping me bring it to life. I'd also like to thank Andrew and Carrie Purcell for the amazing photography and food styling in this book. It was so fun shooting this with you! Truly a dream team.

And lastly to all my amazing friends, family, clients, and community for testing these recipes and listening to my nutrition advice. Your support over the years has meant the world to me. Without you I would not have had the confidence, yet alone the material for this book. Thank you!

Notes

1   Michael Via, "The Malnutrition of Obesity: Micronutrient Deficiencies That Promote Diabetes," *International Scholarly Research Notices*, vol. 2012, Article ID 103472, 8 pages (2012), https://doi.org/10.5402/2012/103472.

2   Felice N. Jacka et al., "Association of Western and Traditional Diets with Depression and Anxiety in Women," *American Journal of Psychiatry*, 167 no. 3 (March 1, 2010): 305–11, https://doi.org/10.1176/appi.ajp.2009.09060881.

3   Eva Selhub, "Nutritional psychiatry: Your brain on food," *Harvard Health Blog*, Harvard Health Publishing, March 26, 2020, https://www.health.harvard.edu/blog/nutritional-psychiatry-your-brain-on-food-201511168626.

4   Thomas Larrieu and Sophie Layé, "Food for Mood: Relevance of Nutritional Omega-3 Fatty Acids for Depression and Anxiety," *Frontiers in Physiology* 9, no. 1047 (August 6, 2018), https://doi.org/10.3389/fphys.2018.01047.

5   Anna Lydia Svalastog et al, "Concepts and definitions of health and health-related values in the knowledge landscapes of the digital society," *Croatian Medical Journal* 58, no. 2 (431–35), https://doi.org/10.3325/cmj.2017.58.431.

6   Elizabeth Lipski, *Digestive Wellness*, 4th ed. (New York: McGraw-Hill, 2011): 155.

7   Joana Araújo, Jianwen Cai, and June Stevens, "Prevalence of Optimal Metabolic Health in American Adults: National Health and Nutrition Examination Survey 2009–2016," *Metabolic Syndrome and Related Disorders* 17, no. 1 (February 8, 2019): 46–52, https://doi.org/10.1089/met.2018.0105.

8   Ariana Chao et al., "Food cravings mediate the relationship between chronic stress and body mass index," *Journal of Health Psychology* 20, no. 6 (June 1, 2015): 721–29, https://doi.org/10.1177/1359105315573448.

9   James L. Wilson, *Adrenal Fatigue: The 21st-Century Stress Syndrome* (Haledon, NJ: Smart Publications).

10   Craig Gustafson, "Bruce Lipton, PhD: The Jump From Cell Culture to Consciousness," *Integrative Medicine: A Clinician's Journal* 16, no. 6 (December 16, 2017): 44–50, https://www.ncbi.nlm.nih.gov/pmc/articles/PMC6438088/.

11   Cynthia A. Daley et al., "A review of fatty acid profiles and antioxidant content in grass-fed and grain-fed beef," *Nutrition Journal* 9, no. 1 (March 10, 2020): 10, https://doi.org/10.1186/1475-2891-9-10.

12   C. J. Lopez-Bote et al., "Effect of free-range feeding on n–3 fatty acid and α-tocopherol content and oxidative stability of eggs," *Animal Feed Science and Technology* 72, nos. 1–2 (1998): 33–40, http://www.centerforfoodsafety.org/files/lopez-bote-1998_32145.pdf.

13   "Research shows eggs from pastured chickens may be more nutritious," Penn State University, June 10, 2010, https://news.psu.edu/story/166143/2010/07/20/research-shows-eggs-pastured-chickens-may-be-more-nutritious.

14   "Added Sugar in the Diet," *The Nutrition Source*, Harvard School of Public Health, https://www.hsph.harvard.edu/nutritionsource/carbohydrates/added-sugar-in-the-diet/.

15   Chika Okada et al., "The Association of Having a Late Dinner or Bedtime Snack and Skipping Breakfast with Overweight in Japanese Women," *Journal of Obesity 2019*, Article ID 2439571 (2019), https://doi.org/10.1155/2019/2439571.

16   Thomas Larrieu and Sophie Layé, "Food for Mood: Relevance of Nutritional Omega-3 Fatty Acids for Depression and Anxiety," *Frontiers in Physiology* 9, no. 1047 (August 6, 2018), https://doi.org/10.3389/fphys.2018.01047.

Index

About the Author

Mia Rigden is a board-certified nutritionist and trained chef with a private nutrition practice in Los Angeles, California. She is the author of *The Well Journal,* and she works with clients globally through one-on-one nutrition coaching and her online courses.

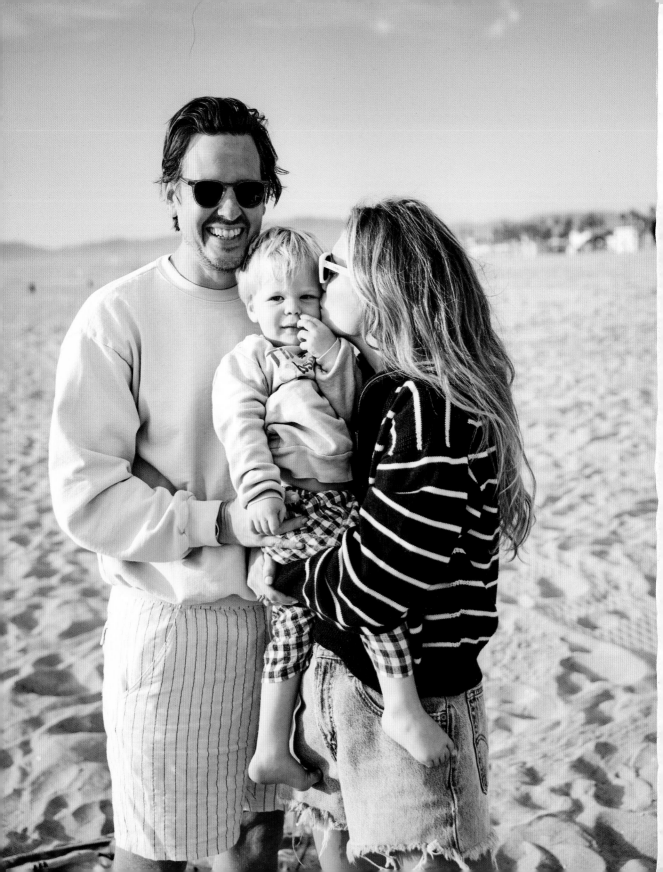